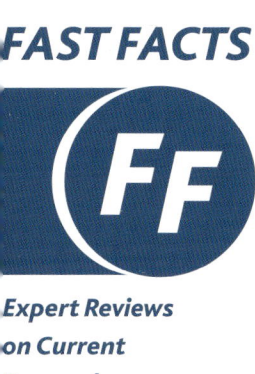

# FAST FACTS

*Expert Reviews on Current Research*

## Highlights 2003–04

Edited by

**Alun H Davies** MA DM FRCS
Reader and Honorary Consultant
Department of Vascular Surgery
Imperial College School of Medicine
Charing Cross Hospital
London, UK

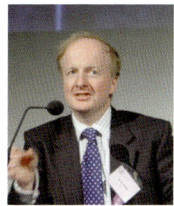

This book is as balanced and as up-to-date as we can make it. Ideas for improvements are always welcome: feedback@fastfacts.com

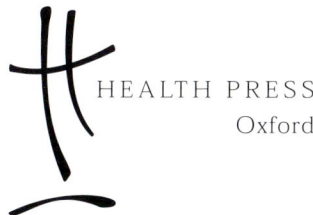

HEALTH PRESS
Oxford

Fast Facts – Vascular Surgery Highlights 2003–04
First published March 2004

© 2004 Health Press Limited
Health Press Limited, Elizabeth House, Queen Street, Abingdon,
Oxford OX14 3JR, UK
Tel: +44 (0)1235 523233
Fax: +44 (0)1235 523238

Book orders can be placed by telephone or via the website.
For regional distributors or to order via the website, please go to:
www.fastfacts.com
For telephone orders, please call 01752 202301 (UK) or
800 538 1287 (North America, toll free).

Fast Facts is a trademark of Health Press Limited.

All rights reserved. No part of this publication may be reproduced, stored in a retrieval system, or transmitted in any form or by any means, electronic, mechanical, photocopying, recording or otherwise, without the express permission of the publisher.

The publisher and the authors have made every effort to ensure the accuracy of this book, but cannot accept responsibility for any errors or omissions.

Registered names, trademarks, etc. used in this book, even when not marked as such, are not to be considered unprotected by law.

A CIP catalogue record for this title is available from the British Library.

ISBN 1-903734-51-7

Davies, AH (Alun)
Fast Facts – Vascular Surgery Highlights 2003–04/
Alun H Davies

Medical illustrations by Dee McLean, London, UK.
Typesetting and page layout by Zed, Oxford, UK.
Printed by Fine Print (Services) Ltd, Oxford, UK.

Printed with vegetable inks on fully biodegradable and recyclable paper manufactured from sustainable forests.

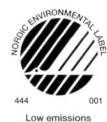

| | |
|---|---|
| Introduction | 5 |
| Hyperhidrosis<br>*Alun H Davies, Clare Ashwin and Nicola Naunton Morgan* | 7 |
| Popliteal entrapment<br>*Luca di Marzo* | 15 |
| Long saphenous vein ablation<br>*Sriram Subramonia and Tim Lees* | 23 |
| External wrapping of the long saphenous vein<br>*Bruno Geier* | 32 |
| Sclerotherapy in venous disease<br>*Jean-Jérôme Guex* | 38 |
| Diagnosis of deep-vein thrombosis<br>*Luis Leon and Nicos Labropoulos* | 45 |
| The role of statins in treating peripheral arterial disease<br>*Judith G Regensteiner* | 53 |
| Regional anesthesia for vascular surgery<br>*Farid Moulla and Avinash Sinha* | 57 |
| Measuring outcomes in vascular surgery<br>*Patrice L Anderson, Annetine Gelijns, Alan J Moskowitz and K Craig Kent* | 64 |
| The effect of renal disease on outcomes of vascular surgery<br>*Peter A McCullough* | 74 |
| Prediction of outcome from ruptured abdominal aortic aneurysm<br>*Fausto Biancari and Tatu Juvonen* | 87 |
| Where is endovascular management of abdominal aortic aneurysm in 2004?<br>*Edward Y Woo and Jeffrey P Carpenter* | 95 |
| Complications of arteriovenous fistula<br>*Michael Walter and Ulrich Boesger* | 102 |
| Blood conservation in thoracic aortic surgery with total cardiopulmonary bypass<br>*Etsuro Suenaga* | 110 |

# Introduction

Readers will, I am sure, find this year's edition of *Vascular Surgery Highlights* as interesting and stimulating as those published in previous years. Among the many topics covered by internationally recognized experts for *Vascular Surgery Highlights* this year, venous disease features prominently, with the techniques of long saphenous vein ablation and external wrapping discussed, two completely different techniques to obtain the same clinical outcome. A further focus is on the outcomes in vascular surgery; this area is becoming increasingly important. To offer patients the best result, we need ways to identify the potential outcomes, firstly to advise patients but also to ensure that accurate comparisons are made when comparing treatment options and individual results from separate institutions.

**Alun H Davies** MA DM FRCS
**Reader and Honorary Consultant, Department of Vascular Surgery**
Imperial College School of Medicine, Charing Cross Hospital, London, UK

# Hyperhidrosis

Alun H Davies MA DM FRCS, Clare Ashwin MBBS and Nicola Naunton Morgan MBBS

Department of Vascular Surgery, Imperial College School of Medicine, London, UK

Hyperhidrosis is a condition of excessive sweat production, which may be generalized to affect the whole body or localized to particular areas, such as the axilla or palms. The consequences can be immensely distressing for a sufferer, causing difficulties with simple tasks such as holding a pen or cup, disruption to personal, social and professional life, and embarrassment. The condition can be secondary to a number of underlying causes, including endocrine disturbance such as thyrotoxicosis or carcinoid tumors, though in many cases no cause can be found. Primary (idiopathic) hyperhidrosis affects around 1% of the population. It may present in childhood,[1] but more commonly does so in adolescence. There is some evidence to suggest that primary hyperhidrosis may have a genetic basis, with 62% of patients in one study reporting a family history, and an autosomal dominant pattern of inheritance has been suggested.[2] Treatments include local topical treatments, anticholinergic therapy, local excision of affected areas, and surgical disruption of the sympathetic chain.

## Pathophysiology

Hyperhidrosis is due to increased secretion of hypotonic fluid from simple tubular eccrine glands situated beneath the dermis, which are innervated by cholinergic fibers from the sympathetic system. Their primary role is in thermoregulation, which is ultimately controlled by the hypothalamus, responding to changes in core body temperature. Anxiety and stress can increase the activity of the eccrine glands via sympathetic drive, though it is thought that sufferers must also have a higher basal rate of secretion.[3]

### Medical treatment

A broad spectrum of treatment options is available, and the choice depends to some extent on the areas affected. Initial treatment is usually topical application to the affected areas. The subjective nature of hyperhidrosis means that the level of intervention is largely dependent on the individual. Psychotherapy has been successful in some cases by reducing anxiety levels, and thus symptoms, to a manageable level. Psychotherapy can also be used as an adjuvant therapy.

**Aluminum chloride preparations** are a popular choice and may have a blocking or astringent action.[4] These treatments are usually effective in 1–3 weeks.[3] They are beneficial in mild to moderate cases, and are relatively inexpensive and easily available. However, long-term use may cause skin irritation, which limits their use in some patients.

**Iontophoresis** is another method that has remained popular, particularly for localized hyperhidrosis of the palms and soles. Electrical current is used to deliver an ionized substance through the skin. Both DC and AC current have been used,[5,6] and successful outcomes have been achieved using tap water, saline and, most successfully, anticholinergics as the ionized agent.[4] Nevertheless, systemic anticholinergic therapy is now seldom used because the large number of side effects limits compliance.

The use of iontophoresis in axillary hyperhidrosis involves application of moistened pads to deliver the electrical current, but this has not been as successful as its use in palmar and plantar regions, where the extremities can be easily bathed.[6] Repeated treatments are required to maintain remission, treatment can be time-consuming, and long-term treatments can cause skin irritation and occasionally burns. Despite this, iontophoresis remains a popular choice for localized palmar or plantar hyperhidrosis.[5,6]

**Botulinum toxin** is an exotoxin produced by *Clostridium botulinum*, which binds irreversibly to cholinergic nerve terminals, preventing acetylcholine release and hence nerve impulse transmission.[7] This biologic action has been put to good use in the treatment of severe localized hyperhidrosis, by blocking sympathetic stimulation of the eccrine glands.[7]

There are three types of botulinum toxin, of which two have been used to date[5,8] and are more commonly known by their proprietary names Botox (type A) and Myobloc (type B). Botox is more established and can achieve remission rates of 2–8 months for axillary sweating and 3–12 months for palmar sweating.[5] The duration of effect is dose-related, and repeated treatments require increasing doses of Botox, possibly due to antibody formation against the type A neurotoxin.[5] As a result, Myobloc has also been investigated as an alternative. Although the injections are more painful due to its acidic nature and it is more expensive, it may play a future role in patients who develop resistance to Botox.

Although Botox has been successful, its use requires careful mapping of the affected area and multiple intradermal injections. These injections can be particularly painful on the palms and soles and may cause temporary weakness of the small muscles of the hand.[3] Regional anesthesia, such as peripheral nerve blocks, has been found to be a more effective method of pain relief than simple local anesthetic creams.[9] With further development of anesthetic techniques, the use of Botox is likely to become more widespread.

## Surgical intervention

Surgical intervention is the only definitive treatment for hyperhidrosis and is used where conservative methods have failed to control symptoms. The latest research has focused on modification of established surgical techniques to minimize their risks, effectively alleviate symptoms, and minimize the development of compensatory hyperhidrosis in other areas. In some cases, this is more of a problem than the initial presenting complaint.[10]

Surgical interventions include:
- local excision of skin, skin and subcutaneous tissue, or with additional surrounding subcutaneous tissue, for axillary hyperhidrosis

- liposuction
- sympathectomy (probably the gold standard).

Complications of local excision are scarring, contractures, hematoma and infection, and skin-flap necrosis.

**Sympathectomy** involves surgical disruption of the sympathetic supply to the eccrine glands of the axilla and palms. It is seldom carried out for plantar hyperhidrosis, as this would require major abdominal surgery and the risk of resultant sexual dysfunction would be high. Multiple open approaches have been established for cervical sympathectomy, including transaxillary and thoracodorsal. In a series of 202 thoracodorsal sympathectomies, a posterior bilateral procedure was as effective as a unilateral staged procedure, and also reduced hospital admissions by half.[11]

For many years, a thoracoscopic approach has been the treatment of choice. The advantages of this technique are minimal tissue disruption and precise visualization of the sympathetic nerves. Complications such as pneumothorax, Horner's syndrome and brachial plexus injuries are also less common. As endoscopic techniques have become more commonplace, the precise surgical methods have been refined and the previous multiportal approach has been replaced by a uniportal or biportal approach.[12]

The basic procedure always involves removal of the second thoracic ganglion and may involve resection of T3 and T4. The stellate ganglion is now left intact, as there is a high risk of Horner's syndrome. The efficacy of thoracoscopic sympathectomy can be further improved by the use of intraoperative monitoring of fingertip temperature or Doppler monitoring of palmar arch blood flow. As the sympathetic fibers are cut, blood supply to the palm will increase by loss of sympathetic vasoconstrictor tone, causing an increase in palmar arch flow and hence fingertip temperature. This correlates well with successful postoperative outcomes.[1]

*Complications.* The development of compensatory hyperhidrosis is the most common complication following sympathectomy. The reasons for this are unclear. It has been suggested that the more extensive the area of skin anhidrosis following surgery, the more severe the resultant compensatory hyperhidrosis.[1] When ganglia are resected, this may result in increased sympathetic traffic through other pathways and thus increased 'compensatory' sweating in other areas. Compensatory hyperhidrosis may mildly affect 86–100% of postoperative patients and increase to severe in 10–40%. In one recent study of 134 patients undergoing a total of 268 sympathectomies, 97% were initially satisfied with their surgery, but, at a mean follow-up of 44 months, 71.9% complained of compensatory hyperhidrosis, and, of these, 19% felt their condition was severe.[13] Of 382 patients who underwent endoscopic thoracic sympathectomy between 1993 and 1998, 120 were followed up at 3 years; 86.4% had some compensatory sweating and 31% rated it as embarrassing, but only 6.3% regretted the operation.[14]

**Sympathotomy** involves the simple disconnection of the second thoracic ganglion from the stellate ganglion rather than removal of the whole ganglion. A very recent case series of 20 procedures in 10 patients reported 100% patient satisfaction with sympathotomy and only mild postoperative hyperhidrosis.[1] The proportion of patients with anhidrosis was also reduced to a mean of 17%, compared with 30% for sympathectomy. In a case-control study of a further 27 patients, there was a significant difference in the proportion of patients with compensatory sweating, which occurred in 45.8% in those who underwent traditional T2 and T3 sympathectomy compared with 16.7% in those who had a selective T2 sympathotomy.[15]

### The role of the nerves of Kuntz
One explanation for the rare failure of sympathectomies or the early recurrence of symptoms involves the nerves of Kuntz. The nerve of Kuntz is a thoracic branch of the first intercostal bundle of nerves (which includes sympathetic fibers) to the brachial plexus. 'Nerves of Kuntz' is a term loosely used to describe fine nerve fibers that arise from T2 and possibly even T3 and T4, bypass the root from which they originate to join neighboring intercostal bundles, and

therefore are not disrupted in sympathectomy and may lead to failure of the procedure.[16] The occurrence of these alternate neural pathways is debatable, with estimates ranging from 0% to 50%. In mid-2003, a single case identification of the nerve of Kuntz was reported in a 19-year-old boy at thoracoscopic sympathectomy.[17] The importance of identifying and disrupting these nerve fibers remains controversial.

### Highlights in hyperhidrosis 2003–04

#### WHAT'S IN?

- Endoscopic clipping techniques
- Reversal procedures to treat compensatory hyperhidrosis
- Botulinum toxin therapy and advances in anesthesia to increase acceptability of repeated injections; possible role in the treatment of compensatory hyperhidrosis
- Full information to the patient of risks and benefits

#### WHAT'S OUT?

- Extensive resection of the sympathetic chain
- Removal of the stellate ganglion
- Multiportal endoscopic techniques

#### WHAT'S NEEDED?

- Clarification of the role of limited sympathectomy to minimize compensatory hyperhidrosis
- Further research into the role of the nerves of Kuntz in early recurrence

## Reversal of sympathectomy

Although endoscopic thoracic sympathectomy is now a simple procedure to perform, it is also an irreversible one after electrocautery or ligation, so it is essential that the patient fully understands the likelihood of success and all the possible outcomes. Occasionally, a patient may be dissatisfied with the outcome because of severe compensatory hyperhidrosis. Recently endoscopic clipping techniques, in which titanium clips can be placed across the nerve to decrease conduction through the sympathetic nerves, have become popular in place of electrocautery or scissors. A compression force of 30 mmHg is needed to inhibit nerve transmission. The procedure can potentially be reversed, though reversal only seems to work if it is attempted soon after surgery and is not guaranteed. A variation called graduated clipping results in slowing of the neural transmissions but not crushing of the nerve fibers, which is theoretically easier to reverse.

A Finnish case study has reported successful open nerve grafting to restore the sympathetic chain following sympathectomy, with subjective relief from compensatory sweating at 1 year and restored sweating in the face and axilla.[18]

### References

1. Atkinson JLD, Fealey RD. Sympathotomy instead of sympathectomy for palmar hyperhidrosis: minimizing postoperative compensatory hyperhidrosis. *Mayo Clin Proc* 2003;78:167–72.

2. Kaufmann H, Saadia D, Polin C et al. Primary hyperhidrosis: evidence for autosomal dominant inheritance. *Clin Auton Res* 2003;13:96–8.

3. Atkins JL, Butler PE. Hyperhidrosis: a review of current management. *Plast Reconstr Surg* 2002;110:222–8.

4. Togel B, Greve B, Raulin C. Current therapeutic strategies for hyperhidrosis: a review. *Eur J Dermatol* 2002;12:219–23.

5. Cheung JS, Solomon BA. Disorders of sweat glands. Hyperhidrosis: unapproved treatments. *Clin Dermatol* 2002;20:638–42.

6. Shimizu H, Tamada Y, Shimizu J et al. Effectiveness of iontophoresis with alternating current in the treatment of patients with *palmoplantar hyperhidrosis*. *J Dermatol* 2003;30:444–9.

7. Campanati A, Penna L, Guzzo T et al. Quality of life assessment in patients with hyperhidrosis before and after treatment with botulinum toxin: results of an open label study. *Clin Ther* 2003;25:298–308.

8. Odderson IR. Hyperhidrosis treated by botulinum A exotoxin. *Dermatol Surg* 1998;24:1237–41.

9. Hayton MJ, Stanley JK, Lowe NJ. A review of peripheral nerve blockade as local anaesthetic in the treatment of palmar hyperhidrosis. *Br J Dermatol* 2003:149:447–51.

10. Connolly M, de Berker D. Management of primary hyperhidrosis: a summary of the different treatment modalities. *Am J Clin Dermatol* 2003;4:681–97.

11. Doblas M, Gutierrez R, Fontcuberta J et al. Thoracodorsal sympathectomy for severe hyperhidrosis: posterior bilateral versus unilateral staged sympathectomy. *Ann Vasc Surg* 2003;17:97–102.

12. Johnson JP, Patel NP. Uniportal and biportal endoscopic thoracic sympathectomy. *Neurosurgery* 2002;51(suppl):79–83.

13. Leseche G, Castier Y, Thabut G et al. Endoscopic transthoracic sympathectomy for upper limb hyperhidrosis: limited sympathectomy does not reduce compensatory sweating. *J Vasc Surg* 2003;37:124–8.

14. Gossot D, Galetta D, Pascal A et al. Long term results of endoscopic thoracic sympathectomy for upper limb hyperhidrosis. *Ann Thorac Surg* 2003;75:1075–9.

15. Yoon do H, Ha Y, Park YG, Chang JW. Thoracoscopic limited T3 sympathocotomy for primary hyperhidrosis: prevention for compensatory hyperhidrosis. *J Neurosurg* 2003;99(suppl):39–43.

16. Singh B, Moodley J, Ramdial PK et al. Pitfalls in thoracoscopic sympathectomy: mechanisms of failure. *Surg Laparosc Endosc Percutan Tech* 2001;11:364–7.

17. Ramsaroop L, Singh B, Moodley J et al. A thoracoscopic view of the nerve of Kuntz. *Surg Endosc* 2003;epub.

18. Milanez de Campos JR, Kauffman P, de Campos Werebe E et al. Quality of life, before and after thoracic sympathectomy: report on 378 operated patients. *Ann Thorac Surg* 2003:76:886–91.

# Popliteal entrapment

### Luca di Marzo MD
Department of Surgery *Pietro Valdoni*, University of Rome *La Sapienza*, Rome, Italy

Popliteal artery entrapment (PAE) was first reported in 1879 by Stuart, a medical student at the University of Edinburgh. During the dissection of an amputated leg of a 64-year-old man, Mr Stuart observed a popliteal artery coursing around the medial head of the gastrocnemius muscle and aneurysmal changes in the popliteal artery distal to the point of external muscular compression.[1] The first case of PAE was surgically treated in 1959, in a 12-year-old boy complaining of claudication after walking 300 m. Surgical exploration revealed an occluded artery with an anomalous course medial to the medial gastrocnemius muscle. The muscle was transected and a successful popliteal artery thromboendarterectomy performed.[2] Since then many case reports have been published, though most have comprised only a small number of patients,[3,4] and were incomplete in detail and patient follow-up.[5]

Both popliteal arterial and venous entrapment are currently considered to be common diseases, together with the functional entrapment first described by Rignault et al.[6] Classification of different types of entrapment, as reviewed by the Popliteal Vascular Entrapment Forum, is reported in Table 1.

## Incidence and demographics

PAE has been described with increasing frequency in the world literature. Gibson et al.[7] observed an incidence of 3.8% in a series of 86 post-mortem limb examinations. Bouhoutsos and Daskalakis[8] treated 33 patients screened out of a series of about 20 000 young vascular patients, an incidence of 0.165%. We detected a similar incidence[9] (2 cases out of 1212 patients studied during a period of 21 months). The real incidence of PAE is still difficult to calculate precisely, because the diagnosis may be difficult at an early stage of the disease and some cases may be dismissed. Taken together,

TABLE 1

**Classification of compressing structures causing popliteal entrapment**

| | |
|---|---|
| Type I | Popliteal artery running medial to the medial head of gastrocnemius |
| Type II | Medial head of gastrocnemius laterally attached |
| Type III | Accessory slip of gastrocnemius |
| Type IV | Popliteal artery passing below popliteal muscle |
| Type V | Primary venous |
| Type VI | Variants |
| Type F | Functional |

however, all the data from the literature indicate that the syndrome is more prevalent than has formerly been appreciated,[10] with more bilateral cases.

PAE usually affects young men (age range 30–40 years) with a male:female ratio of 3.2:1. Entrapment with primary involvement of the popliteal vein (type V) is a rare occurrence occasionally described in the literature.

## Signs and symptoms

Symptoms and signs in patients affected with PAE are extremely variable. A grading scale of symptoms has been proposed (Table 2). In our overall experience, we have observed 26 limbs (45.6%) with class 1 symptoms, 20 (35.1%) with class 2 symptoms, 8 (14.1%) with class 3 symptoms and 1 (1.7%) with class 5 symptoms. Two (3.5%) limbs were asymptomatic. The occurrence of post-stenotic aneurysmal dilatation in PAE is rare (in our series 8 limbs out of 57). The occurrence of moderate-to-severe symptoms thus accounts for less than 16% of all our patients with PAE, which is probably because of the richness of collateral circulation at the knee level and the only rare progression of atherosclerosis in PAE when it is diagnosed at an early stage. For this reason, careful investigation of PAE is recommended in all young patients of either sex presenting with signs and symptoms of

TABLE 2

**Grading of symptoms of popliteal entrapment**

| | |
|---|---|
| Class 0 | Asymptomatic |
| Class 1 | Pain, paresthesia, and cold feet after physical training (sport and heavy work) |
| Class 2 | Claudication (> 100 m) while walking |
| Class 3 | Claudication (< 100 m) while walking |
| Class 4 | Rest pain |
| Class 5 | Necrosis |

pain, paresthesia, cold feet and calf claudication after intensive physical training, to avoid more dramatic clinical presenting symptoms, e.g. arterial atherosclerotic impairment and aneurysmal changes.

It is important to appreciate the similarities between anatomic PAE and the functional form, which some authors describe as the same entity. Rignault et al. first described a form of functional entrapment in an athletic subject who presented with hypertrophied gastrocnemius muscle without an anomalous relationship between the popliteal artery and its surrounding musculotendinous structures.[6] Others have described a compartment syndrome resembling popliteal entrapment in well-conditioned athletes.[11,12]

Patients affected by primarily venous entrapment present symptoms characterized by long-standing calf discomfort (swelling and aching), edema and venous claudication.

## Diagnosis

Signs and symptoms in a young patient should always raise the suspicion of possible PAE, and a careful examination followed by non-invasive evaluation should be performed in each case. The diagnostic evaluation of PAE is an important step in the treatment of this syndrome.[9] Continuous-wave (CW) Doppler ultrasonography with maneuvers that tighten the calf muscles, such as active plantar flexion against resistance, if correctly performed, may allow diagnosis, though false-positive results may occur. The pencil probe should be placed on the posterior tibial artery, avoiding sudden movements during calf muscle contraction, and the examination should be repeated at least three or four times.

Color Doppler scans are a useful tool in diagnosing PAE (Figure 1) and are best performed when the Doppler CW is positive. The popliteal artery should be scanned during calf muscle contraction, when the calf muscles push the artery deep into the popliteal fossa. The scan should be carefully repeated at least three or four times after artery displacement, placing the sample volume correctly in the popliteal artery to avoid false-positive results. We still recommend digital angiography with maneuvers to confirm the diagnosis of PAE before surgical treatment (Figure 2). Computed tomography (CT) and magnetic resonance imaging have been used to detect PAE, simultaneously revealing detailed anatomic information of the popliteal fossa (Figure 3).

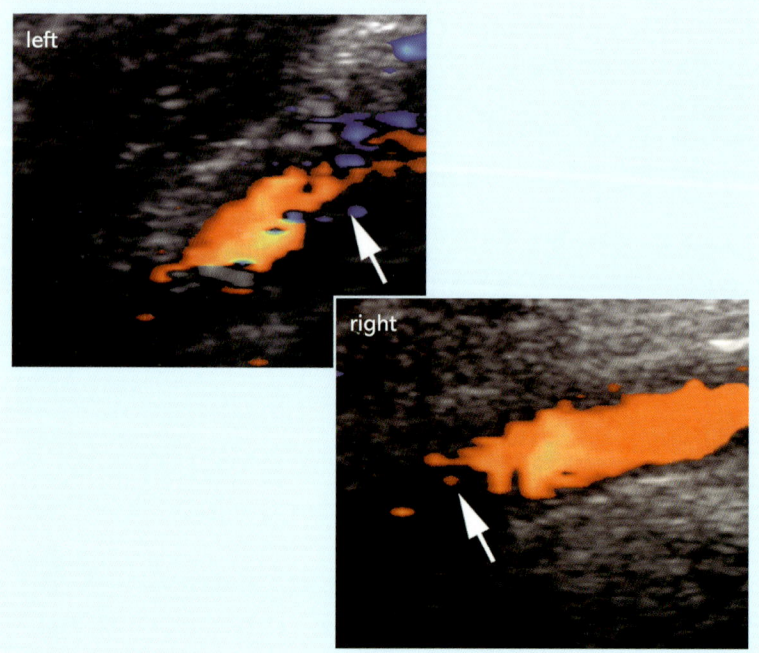

**Figure 1** Color Doppler image recorded during a maneuver in which the calf muscles are tightened.

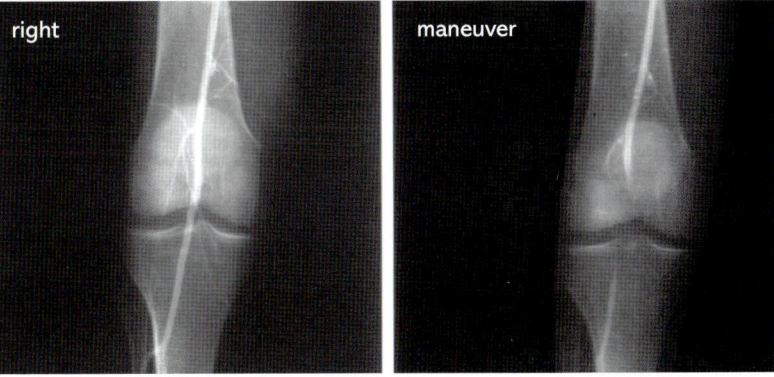

**Figure 2** Arteriography demonstrating popliteal artery entrapment during maneuver.

In our experience, dynamic ascending venography, performed with the patient upright and moderate calf contraction (Figure 4), together with phlebodynamometry with ambulatory venous pressure evaluation, performed separately, are able to diagnose primarily venous entrapment.

## Treatment

Management of the PAE syndrome is surgical, with the exception of cases diagnosed very late with an occluded popliteal artery without

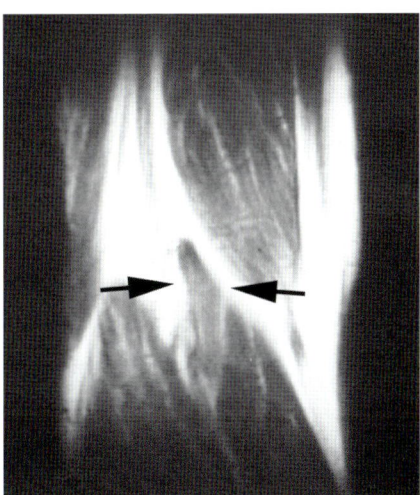

**Figure 3** MRI showing medial gastrocnemius muscle laterally inserted.

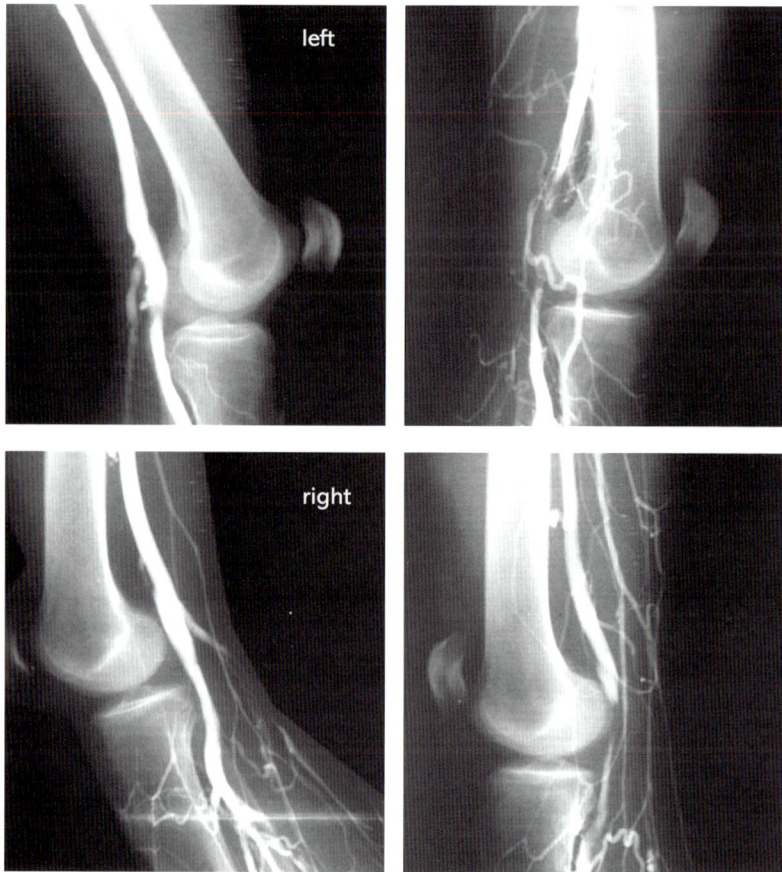

**Figure 4** Venography performed with the patient upright. A compression of the popliteal vein during moderate calf contraction is shown on the right.

aneurysmal changes, in which collateral circulation is considered satisfactory for the patient. Current data encourage attempts to identify patients with PAE at an early stage, when surgical treatment can be limited to musculotendinous section. In our study,[13] we clearly demonstrated that the only parameter influencing long-term outcome is age at presentation. In some of the patients affected with bilateral PAE, arterial reconstruction was required in one limb and musculotendinous section was the treatment of choice in the other. Although the findings could be interpreted as a progressive degeneration of the popliteal artery, it is obvious that, in these cases,

## Highlights in **popliteal entrapment** 2003–04

### WHAT'S IN?

- New classification, including arterial, venous and functional entrapment
- Early diagnosis allowing treatment limited to musculotendinous section with optimal results when compared to arterial reconstruction
- Diagnosis of venous entrapment with ascending venography and ambulatory venous pressure measurements

### WHAT'S OUT?

- Complex classifications
- The idea that arterial, venous and functional entrapment are three different diseases
- Treatment at late stages requiring arterial reconstruction

### WHAT'S CONTROVERSIAL?

- Optimal diagnosis of venous entrapment
- Diagnosis and surgical treatment of functional entrapment

---

time cannot be the only factor to explain the natural history of PAE. Other factors, such as affected side, musculotendinous structures, or dominant limb, were analyzed as possible explanations for the observations, but no statistical associations were found.

Reconstruction of the popliteal artery should be limited in length to the impaired arterial segment, avoiding anastomoses to the tibial vessels whenever possible. The presence of aneurysmal changes does not modify the surgical approach to the popliteal artery, which we always perform through a Z-shaped posterior incision. This is useful when more musculotendinous structures are involved. The medial incision is more anatomic, but does not allow complete exposure of the popliteal fossa, and identification of the compressing structures may be difficult. Autogenous veins should be preferred to prosthetic materials.

**References**

1. Stuart PTA. Note on a variation in the course of the popliteal artery. *J Anat Physiol* 1879;13:162.

2. Hamming JJ. Intermittent claudication at an early age due to anomalous course of the popliteal artery. *Angiology* 1959;10 369–70.

3. Rich NM, Collins GJ, McDonald PT et al. Popliteal vascular entrapment. Its increasing interest. *Arch Surg* 1979;114:1377–84.

4. Collins PS, McDonald PT, Linc RC. Popliteal artery entrapment: an evolving syndrome. *J Vasc Surg* 1989;10:484–90.

5. di Marzo L, Cavallaro A, Sciacca V et al. Natural history of entrapment of the popliteal artery. *J Am Coll Surg* 1994;178:553–6.

6. Rignault DP, Pailler JL, Lunel F. The functional popliteal entrapment syndrome. *Int Angiol* 1985;4:341–3.

7. Gibson MH, Mills JG, Johnson GE, Downs AR. Popliteal entrapment syndrome. *Ann Surg* 1977;185:341–8.

8. Bouhoutsos J, Daskalakis E. Muscular abnormalities affecting the popliteal vessels. *Br J Surg* 1981;68:501–6.

9. di Marzo L, Cavallaro A, Sciacca V et al. Diagnosis of popliteal artery entrapment syndrome: the role of duplex scanning. *J Vasc Surg* 1991;13:434–8.

10. Levien L, Veller MG. Popliteal artery entrapment syndrome: more common than previously recognized. *J Vasc Surg* 1999;30:587–98.

11. Turnipseed WD, Pozniak M. Popliteal entrapment as a result of neurovascular compression by the soleus and plantaris muscles. *J Vasc Surg* 1992;15:285–94.

12. Erdoes LS, Devine JJ, Bernhard VM et al. Popliteal vascular compression in a normal population. *J Vasc Surg* 1994;20:978–86.

13. di Marzo L, Cavallaro A, Mingoli A et al. Popliteal artery entrapment syndrome: the role of early diagnosis and treatment. *Surgery* 1997;122:26–31.

# Long saphenous vein ablation

**Sriram Subramonia** MBBS MS FRCS **and Tim Lees** MBChB FRCS MD
Northern Vascular Centre, Freeman Hospital, Newcastle upon Tyne, UK

Lower extremity varicose veins are one of the commonest disorders presenting to general and vascular surgeons. They may cause prolonged discomfort and disability with impairment in the quality of life.[1] A significant proportion of patients with varicose veins suffer from long saphenous vein incompetence. Surgery is carried out for a range of indications and usually involves saphenofemoral disconnection, stripping of the vein in the thigh and stab avulsions. Surgery itself may cause significant early morbidity, however, and in recent years, less invasive minimal-access techniques have been developed, involving ablation of the long saphenous vein in the thigh without the need for a groin incision or vein stripping. By reducing operative trauma, these techniques might be expected to reduce postoperative morbidity.

Ablation can be achieved with radiofrequency energy, lasers or foam sclerotherapy. Early results are encouraging, but further evidence of their efficacy is required before the techniques become widely accepted in clinical practice. In the UK, the National Institute for Clinical Excellence (NICE) has recently issued a guidance document on the use of radiofrequency ablation,[2] and this technique will be dealt with in some detail in this chapter.

These newer techniques have the potential to cause less morbidity, enabling quicker recovery and return to normal activity, with complication rates and short-term recurrence rates equivalent to conventional surgery. They may arguably reduce long-term recurrence by avoiding a groin wound, which is a potential stimulus for 'neovascularization'. Some of the techniques use costly equipment and demand great skill and experience and good team work, and randomized trials comparing them with conventional surgery to evaluate their clinical efficacy and cost-effectiveness are required before they become established in health care. Currently available safety and efficacy data, however, indicate that these less invasive techniques could offer an alternative to conventional surgery for many patients with long saphenous vein incompetence.

### Radiofrequency ablation

**Principle.** Ablation or luminal obliteration is achieved with radiofrequency resistive heating of the vein wall, controlled by a feedback system for venous wall temperature and impedance and for power consumption by the system. The VNUS Closure system (VNUS Medical Technologies, California) comprises a computer-controlled, bipolar thermal energy generator and catheters with sheathable electrodes. The generator supplies radiofrequency energy at 460 kHz to bipolar catheter electrodes placed intraluminally under duplex ultrasonographic guidance. The high-frequency current passing from the active electrode is converted into heat. This in turn causes venous spasm, with denaturation and irreversible shrinkage of vein wall collagen and intimal destruction. The feedback-controlled heating ensures maximum lumen contraction with preservation of vein integrity. This leads to venous tissue destruction with vein-wall thickening and rapid organization, forming a fibrotic seal of the lumen with minimal thrombus formation. Contraction of the vein wall minimizes the likelihood of recanalization, in contrast to earlier endovenous electrocoagulation methods that relied on thrombus formation.

**Technique.** The entire procedure is performed with duplex ultrasonographic control, either under general anesthesia or with intravenous sedation and local anesthesia.
- The long saphenous vein is accessed percutaneously at the ankle or knee level or via a cut-down at knee level.
- The subcutaneous tissues overlying the long saphenous vein in the thigh are infiltrated with 0.9% saline (or local anesthetic).
- Following positioning of the catheter just distal to the saphenofemoral junction (Figure 1), the leg is elevated and wrapped in an Esmark bandage, and manual compression

applied between the upper limit of this bandage and the saphenofemoral junction to occlude the vein lumen.
- The patient is placed head down.
- The electrodes are unsheathed and wall contact tested by measuring the impedance. The power level, maximum temperature and duration of treatment are then selected.
- Ablation is performed from just below the saphenofemoral junction (usually leaving in circulation the superficial epigastric vein) to the level of the knee, maintaining the temperature of the probe at 85°C, withdrawing the catheter at a rate of approximately 2.5 cm/minute (Figure 2).

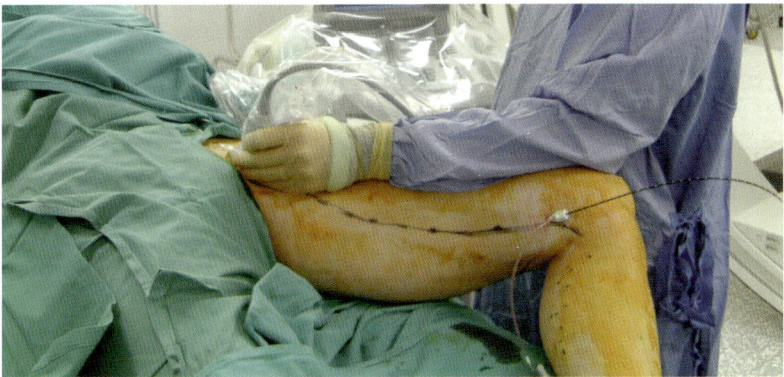

**Figure 1** Catheter tip position just distal to the saphenofemoral junction confirmed by duplex ultrasonography prior to ablation.

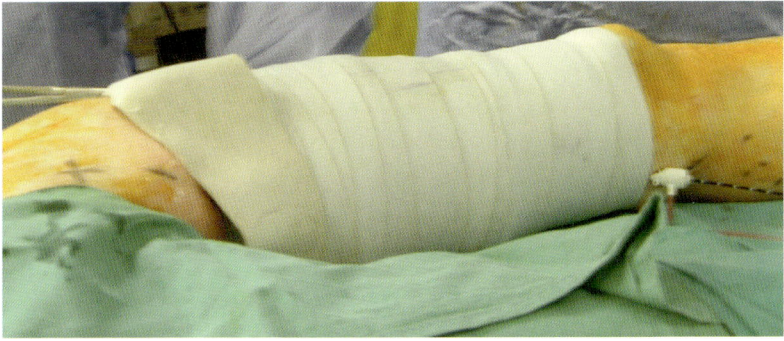

**Figure 2** Ablation in progress with the leg elevated and wrapped in Esmark bandage.

The catheter has a central lumen to facilitate heparinized saline infusion (to avoid thrombus formation on the electrodes) and passage of a guide-wire, if required. Catheters are available in two sizes, 6 Fr and 8 Fr, to allow for obliteration of veins from 2 mm to 12 mm in diameter.

After completion, duplex ultrasonography is used to confirm vein shrinkage. At this stage, there will be minimal flow but not yet complete occlusion of the vein.

**Patient selection.** The primary criterion is duplex ultrasonographic confirmation of long saphenous venous incompetence requiring treatment. Contraindications to radiofrequency ablation are:
- a vein diameter that is less than 2 mm (too small to cannulate) or more than 12 mm (poor impedance) in the supine position
- a very tortuous vein above the knee (unsuitable for catheterization)
- thrombus in the long saphenous vein
- patients with a pacemaker or internal defibrillator.

At present, we do not treat short saphenous vein incompetence because of the risk of sural nerve injury.

**Results.** Early results with VNUS ablation in many centers look promising and are similar to our own experience with this procedure.[3-9] The follow-up period in these studies varied from 6 weeks to 2 years.

*Efficacy.* The immediate vein occlusion rate at 1 week following the procedure is 88–98%,[3,5,6,9] and the continued closure rate at 2 years is 85–90%.[5,6] Doppler ultrasonographically confirmed reflux was observed in about 10% at 2 years.[4,6] Recurrent varicose veins were noted in 7–13% at 2 years[4,6]. Between 94% and 100% of patients were either symptom-free or had significant improvement in symptoms at follow-up,[3-5,9] and patient satisfaction ranged between 92% and 100%.[4-6,8]

Two randomized trials comparing radiofrequency ablation with conventional surgery have shown significantly less pain, lower analgesic requirements, shorter sick leave and quicker restoration of physical function in the radiofrequency group.[8,9]

No studies have yet reported on 5-year follow-up. The 2-year recurrence rate is reported to be 10–15%, which is comparable to that from conventional surgery. Most recurrences were in original anatomic failures, and only a fraction required retreatment. No significant differences in recurrent reflux rates were shown between conventional high ligation and radiofrequency ablation without high ligation. It is postulated that allowing natural drainage of the superficial epigastric vein into the proximal long saphenous vein and avoiding a groin dissection may help prevent the development of collaterals and avoid the stimulus for neovascularization, which is considered the principal cause of recurrence.[10,11] In a recent series, no neovascularization was seen at the groin after radiofrequency ablation at 1-year follow-up.[12]

*Complications.* Minor complications reported include bruising, erythema, hematoma, purpura and clinical phlebitis. More major complications reported are paresthesia (1–19%), thermal injury to skin overlying the vein (0–3%), deep-vein thrombosis (1%) and pulmonary embolism (less than 1%).[3,5,6,9] The incidence of paresthesia seems to be much less when treatment is limited to the thigh and upper leg. Infiltration of saline or local anesthetic around the vein may reduce the risk of paresthesia and skin burns.

*Cost.* Most new technologies are expensive, and radiofrequency ablation is no exception. The additional costs involve the cost of the generator, the catheter (single patient use currently at approximately £550 in the UK per catheter, equivalent to US$1000), the use of duplex ultrasonography, and possibly a longer operating time. A recent randomized trial has indicated, however, that radiofrequency ablation could be cost-saving overall, particularly in the employed group if indirect costs from lost working days are considered.[8]

## Other methods of endovenous long saphenous vein ablation

**Endovenous laser ablation** for long saphenous vein incompetence has also generated much interest in recent years.[13-17] The principle is

## Highlights in long saphenous vein ablation 2003–04

### WHAT'S IN?
- Management of varicose veins in specialist units
- Fully informed consent
- Careful patient selection with duplex ultrasonographic scanning
- A choice of less invasive techniques

### WHAT'S OUT?
- Treatment in units without access to duplex ultrasonographic scanning
- Unsupervised surgery by inexperienced trainees
- Stripping of the long saphenous vein to the ankle

### WHAT'S CONTROVERSIAL?
- Efficacy of new techniques with regard to morbidity, early and late recurrence
- Cost-effectiveness of new techniques
- Applicability of these techniques in the national healthcare system

### WHAT'S NEEDED?
- Prospective, randomized trials comparing less invasive techniques with conventional surgery in relation to benefits, complications, quality of life and costs
- An open mind to the benefit of new techniques
- Skill, shared experiences and team working

similar to that of radiofrequency ablation, with 810 nm diode laser energy delivered via a 600 μm (400–750 μm) laser fiber to heat the vein wall and cause collagen contraction and endothelial denudation, leading to non-thrombotic occlusion. The use of 980 nm and 1064 nm laser energy has also been reported. Results from published series are similar to, if not better than, those of radiofrequency ablation with a lower incidence of complications.[16] The issues of cost and long-term recurrence are similar.

**Foam sclerotherapy.** Sclerotherapy has been in use for many years, but long-term studies have shown superior results for surgical stripping compared with high ligation and sclerotherapy.[18] However, sclerotherapy is still an effective and cheaper treatment option in selected patients.

Studies in recent years have shown the benefits of delivering the sclerosant into the vein as foam mixed with air, with a high immediate success rate, low cost and acceptable complication rate (see page 39).[19,20] The foam bolus reconstitutes in the vein, pushing the blood away and ensuring contact with the endothelium to achieve a sclerosing effect. The reported advantages include:
- better adhesiveness
- echovisibility due to mixing with air
- enhancement of sclerosing power
- reduction of drug doses and concentration.

The safe amount of injected air is 3 mL per session. Various methods of foam production have been described, for example Monfreux, Tessari, Frullini, Cabrera. The outcome at 6 months is encouraging, and long-term results are awaited.[20]

### References

1. Smith JJ, Garratt AM, Guest M et al. Evaluating and improving health-related quality of life in patients with varicose veins. *J Vasc Surg* 1999;30:710–19.

2. National Institute for Clinical Excellence. Radiofrequency ablation of varicose veins. *Interventional Procedure Guidance 8.* London: September 2003.

3. Chandler JG, Pichot O, Sessa C et al. Treatment of primary venous insufficiency by endovenous saphenous vein obliteration. *J Vasc Surg* 2000;34:201–14.

4. Goldman MP, Amiry S. Closure of the greater saphenous vein with endoluminal radiofrequency thermal heating of the vein wall in combination with ambulatory phlebectomy: 50 patients with more than 6-month follow-up. *Dermatol Surg* 2002;28:29–31.

5. Weiss RA, Weiss MA. Controlled radiofrequency endovenous occlusion using a unique radiofrequency catheter under duplex guidance to eliminate saphenous varicose vein reflux: a 2-year follow-up. *Dermatol Surg* 2002;28:38–42.

6. Merchant RF, DePalma RG, Kabnick LS. Endovenous obliteration of saphenous reflux: a multicenter study. *J Vasc Surg* 2002;35:1190–6.

7. Banerjee B, Lees TA, Wyatt MG, Oates C. Radiofrequency ablation of the long saphenous vein in the treatment of lower limb varicose veins. *Phlebology* 2003;18:51.

8. Rautio T, Ohinmaa A, Perala J et al. Endovenous obliteration versus conventional stripping operation in the treatment of primary varicose veins: a randomised controlled trial with comparison of costs. *J Vasc Surg* 2002;35:958–65.

9. Lurie F, Creton D, Eklof B et al. Prospective randomised study of endovenous radiofrequency obliteration (Closure procedure) versus ligation and stripping in a selected patient population (EVOLVeS Study). *J Vasc Surg* 2003;38:207–14.

10. Nyamekye I, Shephard NA, Davies B et al. Clinicopathological evidence that neovascularisation is a cause of recurrent varicose veins. *Eur J Vasc Endovasc Surg* 1998;15:412–15.

11. Jones L, Braithwaite BD, Selwyn D et al. Neovascularisation is the principal cause of varicose vein recurrence: results of a randomised trial of stripping the long saphenous vein. *Eur J Vasc Endovasc* 1996;12:442–5.

12. Fassiadis N, Kianifard B, Holdstock JM, Whiteley MS. Ultrasound changes at the saphenofemoral junction and in the long saphenous vein during the first year after VNUS closure. *Int Angiol* 2002;21:272–4.

13. Bone C. Tratamiento endoluminal de las varices con laser de diodo: estudio preliminary. *Rev Patol Vasc* 1999;5:35–46.

14. Navarro L, Min RJ, Bone C. Endovenous laser: a new minimally invasive method of treatment of varicose veins - preliminary observations using an 810 nm diode laser. *Dermatol Surg* 2001;27:117–22.

15. Gérard JL, Desgranges P, Becquemin JP et al. Peut-on traiter les grandes saphènes variqueuses par laser endoveineux en ambulatoire? Résultats à 1 mois d'une étude de faisabilité sur 20 patients traités en salle de consultation. *J Mal Vasc* 2002;27:222–5.

16. Min RJ, Khilnani N, Zimmet SE. Endovenous laser treatment of saphenous vein reflux: long-term results. *J Vasc Interv Radiol* 2003;14:991–6.

17. Chang C, Chua J. Endovenous laser photocoagulation (EVLP) for varicose veins. *Lasers Surg Med* 2002;31:257–62.

18. Rutgers PH, Kitslaar PJ. Randomized trial of stripping versus high ligation combined with sclerotherapy in the treatment of the incompetent greater saphenous vein. *Am J Surg* 1994;168:311–15.

19. Min RJ, Navarro L. Transcatheter duplex ultrasound-guided sclerotherapy for treatment of greater saphenous vein reflux: a preliminary report. *Dermatol Surg* 2000;26:410–14.

20. Frullini A, Cavezzi A. Sclerosing foam in the treatment of varicose veins and telangiectases: history and analysis of safety and complications. *Dermatol Surg* 2002;28:11–15.

# External wrapping of the long saphenous vein: a treatment option in varicose vein surgery

**Bruno Geier** MD

Division of Vascular Surgery, Ruhr University Bochum, Germany

The classic operative treatment for long saphenous vein (LSV) insufficiency consists of stripping of the insufficient vein from the saphenofemoral junction (SFJ) to below the knee or to the ankle. Performed correctly, this is a safe and effective procedure that achieves good short- and long-term results and is still the treatment of choice for most patients with LSV insufficiency. However, one disadvantage of this technique is the loss of the LSV as a potential bypass graft. Furthermore, the distal incisions on the lower leg or the ankle carry the potential danger of saphenous nerve injury, which can result in persistent paresthesia.[1,2] This has led to the development of operations that allow treatment of the reflux without stripping of the LSV. One of these techniques is external valvuloplasty of the SFJ. The principle of the operation is to restore the function of the vein valves in the SFJ by extraluminal wrapping of the dilated LSV, thereby reducing its diameter and bringing the vein cusps together. The technique was first presented in 1988 by Jessup and Lane, who used a preformed Dacron (polyester) cuff (Venocuff).[3] Since 1995 we have been treating selected patients with LSV insufficiency with external wrapping of the saphenofemoral junction using a home-made Dacron cuff.

## Patient selection and operative technique

A thorough and careful examination of the SFJ and the LSV with duplex ultrasonography is crucial in selecting patients for external wrapping. The procedure can be considered for patients with reflux at the SFJ if:
- ultrasonography demonstrates intact and mobile cusps of the terminal and subterminal valve of the LSV
- the diameter of the LSV at the SFJ does not exceed 12 mm.

A diameter of less than 5 mm is regarded as a contraindication to valvuloplasty as it indicates a primary valve defect as the cause of the reflux.[4] In addition, hemodynamically significant perforator insufficiencies at the thigh level as well as gross tortuosity and pronounced aneurysmal degeneration along the course of the LSV are arguments against external wrapping.

The operation can be performed through a small (3–4 cm) incision in the groin. The SFJ is dissected out and all side branches are transsected and ligated. The anterior wall of the deep vein is also exposed 1–2 cm proximal to the origin of the LSV. We then use a rectangle of Dacron to create a cuff which is placed circumferentially around the SFJ, thereby reducing the diameter of the LSV and rendering the valves competent (Figure 1). To achieve the same result, Lane et al.[5] use a preformed, commercially available cuff which allows the defined reduction of the LSV diameter to 4.4, 5.5 or 6.5 mm (Figure 2). To assess the competency of the valve after the valvuloplasty, a strip test of the LSV can be performed or a distal side branch can be used to test for persisting reflux while the patient is performing a Valsalva maneuver or, if the operation is done under general anesthesia, positive airway pressure is applied.

Immediately after the operation the leg is wrapped with elastic bandages; these are replaced with compression stockings on the first postoperative day. After 6 weeks the patient is re-examined, and any persisting varicose side branches or perforating vein insufficiencies seen with duplex ultrasonography are treated with sclerotherapy.

## Results

Lane et al. have recently published the results of their extensive experience with external valvuloplasty of the SFJ, which consisted of 1516 cases in 15 years.[5] They followed up their 107 patients with duplex ultrasonography and found a competent SFJ in 90% of cases after a mean 4.8 years. The mean diameter of the LSV distal to the cuff decreased from 7.6 to 4.9 mm, and the diameter of the LSV at the knee decreased from 6.9 to 3.7 mm. The rate of recurrence was 9% at 4.9 years.

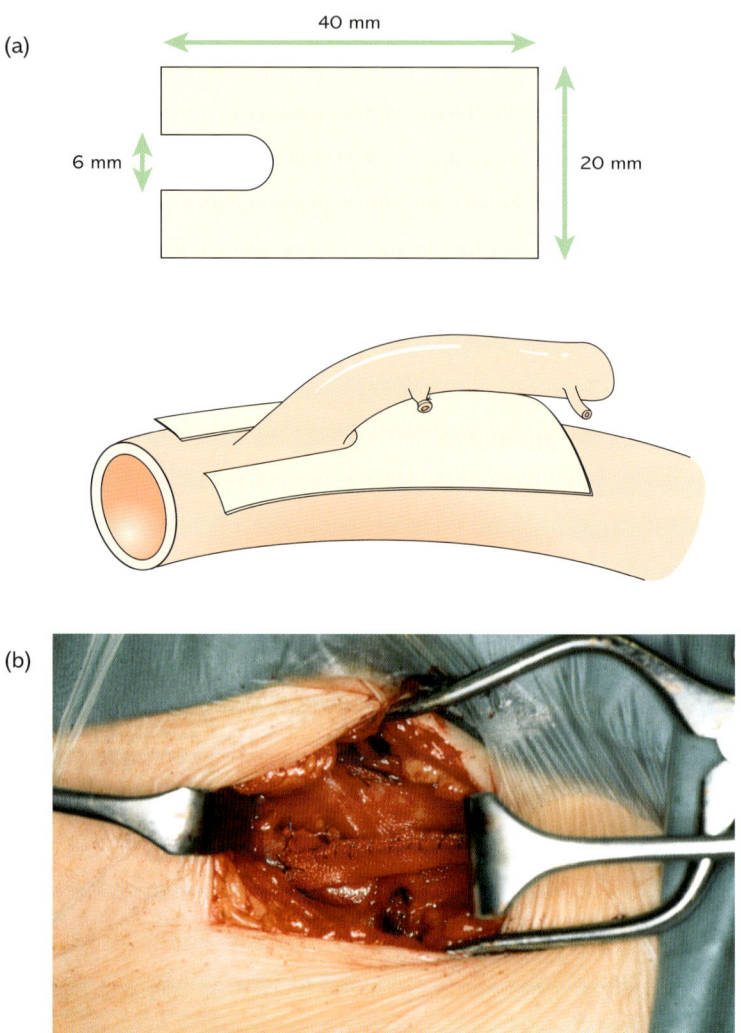

**Figure 1** (a) Size and placement of the Dacron cuff. (b) Intraoperative view after completion of the valvuloplasty.

We found similar results in a group of 50 patients with 54 valvuloplasties, who were followed up after 54 months.[6] The competence rate was 89%, the diameter of the LSV was reduced by a mean of 3 mm and the venous refill time was reduced by a mean of 5 seconds. The rate of symptomatic recurrence was 18.5%. The

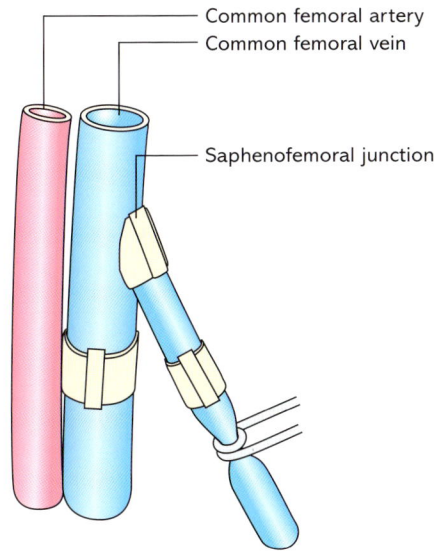

**Figure 2** Venocuff used by Lane et al.[5]

only other study with a similarly long follow-up of 52 months has been published by Zamboni et al., who report a competency rate of 94% and a recurrence rate of 12%.[7]

Several reports of external valvuloplasty of the LSV with a shorter follow-up of 1–2 years describe good results in terms of valve competency, LSV patency and recurrence rate.[8–10] In addition, Schanzer and Skladany found a significantly higher rate of thrombotic occlusion of the LSV after high ligation than after external wrapping of the SFJ.[11]

## Conclusion

External wrapping of the LSV is a safe and cosmetically favorable procedure which is accepted very well by patients and delivers 5-year results comparable with those of stripping in terms of relief of symptoms and recurrence rate. The available data show that even after 5 years the varicose degeneration of the LSV is prevented or even reversed. The key to achieving good results is careful patient selection, the best indications being mild-to-moderate LSV incompetence and incompetent anterior or lateral accessory systems. The combination of

## Highlights in **external wrapping of the long saphenous vein: a treatment option in varicose vein surgery** 2003–04

### WHAT'S IN?
- Careful duplex ultrasound examination to choose the operative treatment for each individual patient with varicose veins
- Combination of valve-repairing surgery with sclerotherapy of smaller side branches and perforators

### WHAT'S OUT?
- External wrapping of the long saphenous vein (LSV) in cases of extensive varicose degeneration
- High ligation of the saphenofemoral junction.

### WHAT'S NEEDED?
- Long-term follow-up
- Randomized studies comparing external wrapping of the LSV and stripping

external wrapping of the LSV with sclerotherapy of perforators and side branches allows a minimally invasive approach to varicose veins while still adhering to the principle of eliminating the reflux at its point of origin. However, since only a relatively small number of patients with varicose veins are candidates for this technique – about 15% in our patient population – it is clearly not a replacement for the classic stripping operation, just an alternative in selected cases. Furthermore, long-term results with follow-up of 10 years or more are needed before a final conclusion about this procedure can be made.

## References

1. Mildner A, Hilbe G. Complications in surgery of varicose veins. *Zentralbl Chir* 2001;126:543–5.

2. Morrisson C, Dalsing M. Signs and symptoms of saphenous nerve injury after greater saphenous vein stripping: prevalence, severity, and relevance for modern practice. *J Vasc Surg* 2003;38:886–90.

3. Jessup G, Lane RJ. Repair of incompetent venous valves: a new technique. *J Vasc Surg* 1988;8:569–75.

4. Reuther T, Nordmeier R, El Gammal C et al. Diameter of the long saphenous vein at the saphenofemoral junction comparing normal and primary varicose veins. *Phlebologie* 1999;28:48–52.

5. Lane RJ, Cuzzilla ML, Coroneos JC. The treatment of varicose veins with external stenting to the saphenofemoral junction. *Vasc Endovasc Surg* 2002;36:179–92.

6. Geier B, Voigt I, Marpe B et al. External valvuloplasty in the treatment of greater saphenous vein insufficiency: a five-year follow up. *Phlebology* 2003;18:137–42.

7. Zamboni P, Marcellino MG, Capelli M et al. Saphenous vein sparing surgery: principles, techniques and results. *J Cardiovasc Surg (Torino)* 1998;39:151–62.

8. Corcos L, Peruzzi GP, Romeo V et al. External valvuloplasty of the saphenofemoral junction. *Phlebologie* 1991;44:497–508.

9. Ik Kim D, Boong Lee B, Bergan JJ. Venous hemodynamic changes after external banding valvuloplasty with varicosectomy in the treatment of primary varicose veins. *J Cardiovasc Surg (Torino)* 1999;40:567–70.

10. Incandela L, Belcaro G, Nicolaides AN et al. Superficial vein valve repair with a new external valve support (EVS). The IMES (International Multicenter EVS Study). *Angiology* 2000;51:39–52.

11. Schanzer H, Skladany M. Varicose vein surgery with preservation of the saphenous vein: a comparison between high ligation-avulsion versus saphenofemoral banding-valvuloplasty-avulsion. *J Vasc Surg* 1994;20:684–7.

# Sclerotherapy in venous disease

**Jean-Jérôme Guex** MD FACPH

Phlebology and Vascular Laboratory, Nice, France

Conventional sclerotherapy has been used for decades in the treatment of varicose disease. However, because of the high rate of recanalization and improper assessment criteria,[1] it is considered disappointing in the treatment of large varicose veins and is limited to the treatment of small varicose veins.

Over the last few years, the use of ultrasonography to guide the injections and the use of foam instead of liquid sclerosing agents have completely modified the technique. Short-to-mid-term results seem extremely promising[2] and the technique is simple, mild, ambulatory, safe and cost-effective.

Foam ultrasound-guided sclerotherapy is a new and reliable alternate treatment for varicose veins, and should become part of the vascular surgeon's toolkit.

## The search for the best primary treatment of large varicose veins

The aim of all treatments for varicose disease is to suppress one or all of the following:
- sources of reflux (incompetent junctions and perforators)[3]
- long refluxes (trunks within the saphenous fascias)
- varicose reservoirs (varicose networks outside the saphenous fascias).

Pathophysiology and experience dictate that treatment should be in the order given. Current techniques for treatment are:
- surgery (flush ligation, stripping and stab avulsion)
- ambulatory phlebectomy (Muller's technique)
- endovascular techniques (radiofrequency, laser, foam sclerotherapy).

Since these techniques differ in so many points and since no universal assessment criteria have been found, no consensus for determining the best treatment has been obtained so far. Completely different approaches according to individual physician's and patient's preferences can provide a completely satisfactory response. Finally, the techniques are evolving faster than the disease itself, which explains why there have been no long-term studies.

## Advantages of duplex guidance of sclerosing injections

Duplex-guided access obviously enhances accuracy, avoids extravenous injections and provides immediate and secondary information on the efficacy of the injections. The effects of the sclerosing agent on the endothelium are immediately visible, with formation of a thin white line on the venous wall. The observation of a venous spasm is also very common and has been considered predictive of success. The technique requires care and training, but accessing 3 mm veins 3 cm deep is easily feasible. A black-and-white B-mode machine is sufficient; color and pulsed Doppler are optional. However, a linear high-frequency probe (7.5–10 MHz) is necessary.

## Advantages of foam sclerotherapy

Foam is an excellent contrast medium for duplex ultrasonography. It allows perfect control of both the injection and the progression of the agent in the veins. Foam does not mix much with blood; thus the concentration of sclerosing agent in contact with the endothelium is almost constant around and along the part of the vein filled with foam. This ensures a more even and powerful effect. Foam can be massaged – manually or with the probe – to the desired veins. In very large veins, it is important to remember that foam floats and that, if no spasm occurs, only the 'upper' wall of the vein will be in contact with the foam and therefore treated.

## How to make foam

Tessari has described a simple technique to produce foam using two 5 mL syringes and a three-way stopcock.[2] Our current method is to introduce gas and liquid into different syringes; foam is obtained after 15–20 alternate passages between syringes. Provensis has a ready-made microfoam in trials (using Cabrera et al.'s technique[4]), and an automated foaming machine is being tested in a study sponsored by the French Society of Phlebology.

## How to carry out duplex-guided injections

The procedure (Table 1) involves:
- holding the duplex probe and putting the needle in the vein at the same time
- aspirating to cross-check for blood reflux
- preparing foam
- injecting the foam to fill the vein
- massaging the foam to the desired part of the varicose network, injecting more foam if necessary.

An open vein access is much more convenient than injecting with a needle attached to the syringe, even with an assistant. The usual devices used are: a winged infusion set (see Figure 1), sufficient in 90% of cases, a needle with connector, microcatheters and long catheters (internal or Seldinger).

TABLE 1

- Place butterfly, needle or catheter into vein under duplex guidance; let blood reflux freely into hose and drip into disposable tray.
- Attach needle to skin with adhesive tape.
- Prepare foam according to Tessari's technique. (We use 1 mL 0.5–3% Polidocanol plus 3 mL air.)
- Check free reflux (free bleeding), then attach syringe to hose.
- Place duplex probe over needle. Inject 0.1 mL foam; check for intraluminal bubbles on duplex.
- Inject as much foam as necessary to fill the whole vein to be treated. Massage with the probe to get foam to the desired veins.
- Check endothelial lesion and venous spasm.
- Remove the needle. Apply a cottonwool ball, adhesive compression tape, compressive pad (optional) and grade-2 thigh-high compression stockings.
- Recommend walking.
- Review the patient (duplex ultrasonography) after 1 week.

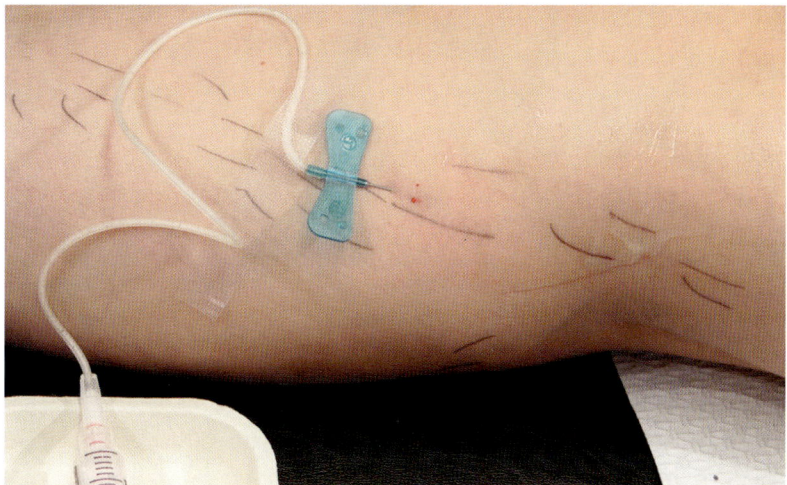

Figure 1. Foam injection.

## What to inject and how much

Usual detergent sclerosing agents (e.g. Polidocanol, Sotradecol) are able to foam. The liquid:gas ratio ranges from 1:3 to 1:6 according to authors. Air is the most commonly used gas, although several authors have proposed using oxygen, carbon dioxide, nitrogen or nitrogen dioxide. Many authors recommend 3% foam for 'large' trunk vessels and 1% for smaller ones. A study is currently in progress in France to determine the difference in effect between 3% and 1% Polidocanol.

The maximum volume of foam varies according to authors, ranging between 5 and 30 mL. Some authors recommend injecting foam until no blood refluxes into the catheter.

## Complications

Ultrasound guidance and use of foam should ensure there is no intra-arterial injection; nevertheless, several cases of necrosis have been reported. Allergy to foam is non-specific. Deep-vein thrombosis has been observed. The incidence is still unclear but is probably less than 1% – a registry has been started in France to provide more information. Superficial thrombophlebitis is observed in 10% of cases but is an excessive reaction rather than a real complication.

> ### Highlights in **sclerotherapy in venous disease** 2003–04
>
> **WHAT'S IN?**
> - Ultrasound-guided open vein access
> - Foam injections
>
> **WHAT'S OUT?**
> - Direct injections with attached syringe and needle
> - Liquid sclerosing agents in trunk veins and large veins
>
> **WHAT'S CONTROVERSIAL?**
> - The prognostic value of the venous spasm
> - The ideal composition of the foam
>
> **WHAT'S NEEDED?**
> - Criteria to assess and compare the results of completely different techniques such as foam sclerotherapy and surgery
> - Mid- and long-term results

Visual gray veil and migraine (possibly equivalent) have been reported,[5] and various explanations have been given. We believe that there is relationship with the volume and density of the foam.

### Results

The superior efficacy of foam compared with liquid has been demonstrated.[6] The overall efficacy of foam injections in great and small saphenous trunk veins is 65% occlusion at the first injection and 95% occlusion after three injections.

The minimum length to be treated in a session is a 'limb-segment' length of varicose vein. The maximum diameter that can be treated by foam sclerotherapy is unknown. Varicose vein wall dysplasia increases with time, and age seems to facilitate the sclerosing process; therefore very large veins can be treated in elderly patients.

### Are liquid sclerosing agents still useful?

Liquid sclerosing agents are still useful in the treatment of small varices, reticular veins and telangiectasias. In these veins, the use of foam is debatable and its instability is a drawback. Therefore the old technique is used.[7,8]

### Are there other indications for foam sclerotherapy?

Foam sclerotherapy has been used in the treatment of venous malformations.[9] In association with coil embolization, it is also becoming popular for the treatment of dilated gonadal and/or hypogastric veins in pelvic congestion syndrome and varicocele.[10]

### References

1. Guex J-J, Isaacs MN. Comparison of surgery and ultrasound guided sclerotherapy for treatment of saphenous varicose veins: must the criteria for assessment be the same? *Int Angiol* 2000;19:299–302.

2. Cavezzi A. Sclérothérapie à la mousse (méthode de Tessari): étude multicentrique. *Phlébologie* 2002;55:149–54.

3. Guex J-J. Ultrasound guided sclerotherapy for perforating veins. *Hawaii Med J* 2000;59:261.

4. Cabrera J, Cabrera J Jr, Garcia Olmedo MA. Treatment of varicose long saphenous veins with sclerosant in microfoam form: long term outcomes. *Phebology* 2000; 15:19–23.

5. Benigni JP, Ratinahirana H. Mousse de polidocanol et migraine à aura. *Phlébologie* 2003;56:289–91.

6. Hamel-Desnos C, Desnos C, Wollmann JC et al. Evaluation of the efficacy of Polidocanol in the form of foam compared with liquid form in sclerotherapy of the greater saphenous vein: initial results. *Dermatol Surg* 2003;29:1170–5.

7. Guex J-J. Microsclerotherapy. *Semin Dermatol* 1993;12(2): 129–34.

8. Guex J-J. Indications for the sclerosing agent Polidocanol®. *J Dermatol Surg Oncol* 1993;19: 959–61.

9. Cabrera J Jr, Garcia-Olmedo MA, Dominguez JA, Mirasol JA. Microfoam: a novel pharmaceutical dosage form for sclerosants. In: Henriet JP, ed. *Foam Sclerotherapy State of the Art*. Paris: Editions Phlébologiques Françaises, 2002.

10. Leal-Monedero J, Zubicoa Ezpeleta S. The role of sclerosing foam in the treatment of pelvic congestion syndrome. In: Henriet JP, ed. *Foam Sclerotherapy State of the Art*. Paris: Editions Phlébologiques Françaises, 2002.

# Diagnosis of deep-vein thrombosis

**Luis Leon** MD and **Nicos Labropoulos** MD PhD DIC RVT

Division of Vascular Surgery, Loyola University Medical Center, Illinois, USA

Deep-vein thrombosis (DVT) and pulmonary embolism (PE) combined are responsible for a large number of hospital admissions and for more than 50 000 deaths every year.[1] The clinical diagnosis of DVT is inaccurate: it has low sensitivity because many thrombi are asymptomatic, and low specificity because many other pathologies can mimic its signs and symptoms. Of those presenting with suggestive symptomatology, only up to one-third will actually have the disorder.[2] In our own center, the prevalence of DVT among patients referred with clinical suspicion is 14%,[3] a figure in agreement with the preliminary analysis of a multicenter study we are conducting. Several methods are available for diagnosis of DVT, including:

- ascending venography
- duplex ultrasonography
- magnetic resonance venography
- computed tomographic (CT) venography
- D-dimer and pretest probability.

## Ascending venography

Although this is the gold standard for the diagnosis of DVT, it has important clinical and methodologic limitations. It is invasive and has significant morbidity, particularly when used for systematic screening of patients in a clinical study. It has a 1.3% risk of causing DVT[4] and does not show other conditions that may explain the patient's symptomatology, such as Baker's cysts, hematomas, enlarged lymph nodes, musculoskeletal injuries, aneurysms and tumors.[5] Alternative, safer, non-invasive methods have significantly reduced the usage of ascending venography, and its quality varies significantly in different centers because of the consequent lack of training.

Radionuclide venography uses technetium-labeled macro-aggregated albumin injected into a foot vein. It has poor resolution for calf DVT, and is unable to distinguish intrinsic from extrinsic compression and occlusive from non-occlusive thrombus. Radiolabeled substances such as fibrinogen, albumin, red blood cells and platelets have been considered for the diagnosis of DVT using scintigraphy, with suboptimal results. Concerns regarding blood-borne disease transmission has restricted use of this method.

**Duplex ultrasonography**
Duplex ultrasonography (DUS) combines Doppler and B-mode ultrasonography. The former yields data regarding spontaneous and phasic venous flow and valve function, and the latter analyzes the vein wall and lumen in real time and can visualize intraluminal thrombus. It has replaced venography as the method of choice for the diagnosis of DVT.

DUS is routinely performed with medium-frequency, linear-array transducers of 4–7 MHz. The limbs of obese patients, the pelvic veins and inferior vena cava are examined with low-frequency phased or curvilinear-array transducers of less than 4 MHz. All veins from the groin to the ankle are examined using compression on B-mode, imaging by color flow, and Doppler signals with augmentation maneuvers. The technique for both the proximal (femoropopliteal veins) and calf veins (posterior tibial, peroneal, gastrocnemial and soleal veins) has been described in detail previously.[3,5] The great and small saphenous veins are identified and examined similarly. The pelvic veins and inferior vena cava are selectively examined. Continuous common femoral vein flow with absent or limited phasicity by Doppler, poor distal common femoral vein augmentation, asymmetric common femoral vein waveforms and bilateral leg symptoms with normal lower extremity DUS mandate their evaluation.

- DUS is negative if complete approximation of the near and far vein walls during compression (Figure 1) or complete color filling of the lumen without defects is visualized.

- DUS is positive if a vein is partially or non-compressible, if echogenic material is seen within the vein, or if a filling defect on color imaging or absence of Doppler signal is identified (Figure 2).

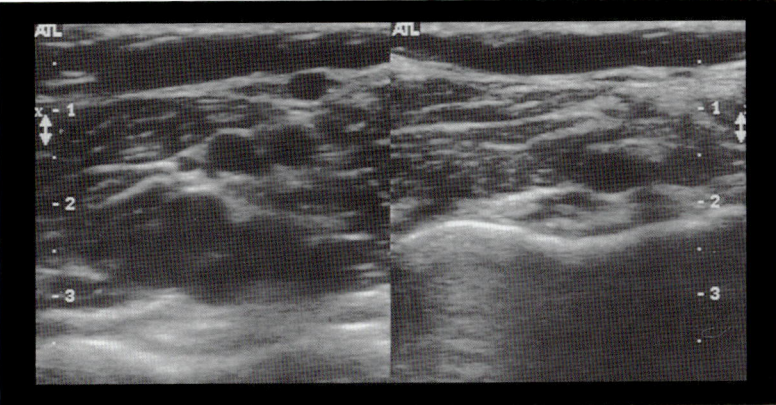

**Figure 1** Cross-sectional view of the popliteal fossa. The popliteal vein is duplicated. The two veins in the middle are the medial gastrocnemial. The one on top is the small saphenous vein. During compression, all veins are collapsed, as shown on the right of the split screen.

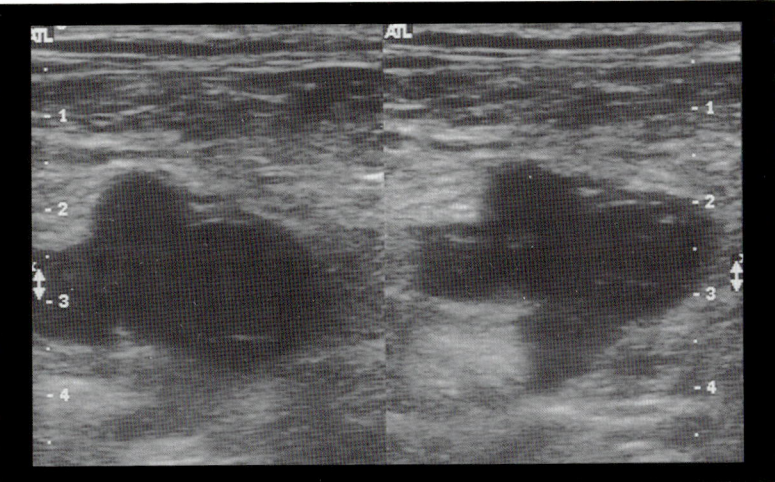

**Figure 2** Acute DVT in the common femoral vein at the level of the femoral artery bifurcation. The vein is distended and non-compressible, as seen on the split screen. Note the presence of echogenic material within the vein lumen.

The diagnostic criteria for acute and chronic thrombosis are shown in Table 1. It is important to distinguish between chronic and recurrent DVT. The latter may occur in a previously affected vein, in a different location that was not previously involved, or in the contralateral limb. The location and size of the new thrombus should be compared with those seen in prior DUS for its diagnosis. An increase of more than 2 mm in the compressed lumen of a previously thrombosed vein has been suggested to be diagnostic of recurrent DVT, but this requires further confirmation.[6,7]

A great advantage of DUS is that it can diagnose other pathologies that could explain the patients' symptoms and may alter their management. Important findings include aneurysms or pseudoaneurysms, hemorrhage and tumors.

TABLE 1

**Diagnostic criteria to differentiate between acute and chronic DVT**

| Criterion | Acute | Chronic |
|---|---|---|
| Vein size | Distended | Reduced; sometimes vein cannot be traced for its entire length by DUS |
| Collateral vessels | Not usually seen | Often found around obstructed segments |
| Lumen echogenicity | Echolucent or of intermediate echogenicity; brightness is less than in neighboring tissues | Old thrombus and/or scar tissue often produces bright echoes within the lumen |
| Lumen characteristics | The lumen is non- or partially compressible | Partial recanalization with filling defects and reflux may be present |
| Wall characteristics | Thin and smooth | In fully recanalized veins, wall thickening with luminal reduction may be seen |

## Magnetic resonance venography

High-resolution images are produced when radiofrequency pulses are applied to a patient within a magnetic field. Excellent sensitivities and specificities have been reported, especially for the inferior vena cava and pelvic veins. Compared with standard venography, magnetic resonance venography:
- is less invasive
- is associated with lower morbidity
- may identify other soft-tissue pathology.[8]

However, it does not offer significant advantages over DUS. It costs more, is cumbersome, cannot be used with metallic implants or claustrophobic patients, requires a lot of time, and is not widely available. Therefore, this technique should be used as a complementary test to DUS.

## CT venography

CT venography of the legs and abdominal veins is usually combined with CT angiography of the pulmonary arteries to allow a complete examination of venous thromboembolism.[9] CT venous phase imaging at the time of CT pulmonary angiography gave results comparable with DUS in the evaluation of femoropopliteal DVT in 71 patients with suspected PE.[10] CT is very good in evaluation of the pelvic veins and inferior vena cava, but there are no studies showing its accuracy in the calf veins. Obvious disadvantages include:
- invasiveness
- inability to be performed at the bedside
- cost
- the need for ionizing radiation and iodinated contrast material.

## D-dimer and pretest probability

D-dimer is a degradation product of cross-linked fibrin; its levels are elevated in almost all patients with a thromboembolic event. Several other states, however, such as advanced age, infection, inflammation, vasculitis, pregnancy, trauma, cancer and the postoperative state, are associated with high D-dimer levels,[2,11] and

## Highlights in **deep vein thrombosis** 2003–04

### WHAT'S IN?

- Accurate diagnosis of DVT so that treatment can be tailored accordingly
- Use of DUS as the method of choice for diagnosis
- The combination of pretest probability and D-dimer testing for acute DVT screening in the outpatient setting

### WHAT'S OUT?

- Reliability of the diagnosis of DVT solely based on clinical grounds
- Standard venography as the method of choice for the diagnosis of acute DVT and as the gold standard tool for comparison in clinical trials
- Radionuclide venography and scintigraphy as first-line imaging modalities

### WHAT'S CONTROVERSIAL?

- The increasing role of magnetic resonance venography for the diagnosis of DVT in the acute setting

### WHAT'S NEEDED?

- Education of healthcare professionals about the management of venous thromboembolism, which may improve its prevention and early diagnosis its use is limited in those conditions. A recent trial has shown that pretest probability, either empirically or using a score system with stratification into risk groups, combined with D-dimer testing, reduces the need for initial and supplementary imaging in the outpatient setting.[11] In patients who are clinically unlikely to have DVT, a prevalence of 5% has been reported using the D-dimer test. A negative D-dimer test can rule out DVT without additional imaging, because it has a high negative predictive value. In patients who are likely to have DVT, D-dimer testing will also reduce the number of DUS procedures required, but it is unknown whether it is cost-effective as the prevalence of DVT is at least 30% in this group.[11] Given its low positive predictive value, patients with a positive D-dimer test need further confirmatory testing and should undergo urgent DUS.

### References

1. Peterson KL. Acute pulmonary thromboembolism: has its evolution been redefined? *Circulation* 1999;99:1280–3.

2. Bockendstedt P. D-dimer in venous thromboembolism. *N Engl J Med* 2003;349:1203–4.

3. Labropoulos N, Webb KM, Kang SS et al. Patterns and distribution of isolated calf deep vein thrombosis. *J Vasc Surg* 1999;30:787–91.

4. Hull R, Hirsh J, Sackett DL et al. Clinical validity of a negative venogram in patients with clinically suspected venous thrombosis. *Circulation* 1981;64:622–5.

5. Labropoulos N, Leon M, Kalodiki E et al. Colour flow duplex scanning in suspected acute deep vein thrombosis: experience with routine use. *Eur J Vasc Endovasc Surg* 1995;9:49–52.

6. Prandoni P, Lensing AW, Bernardi E et al. The diagnostic value of compression ultrasonography in patients with suspected recurrent deep vein thrombosis. *Thromb Haemost* 2002;88:402–6.

7. Prandoni P, Cogo A, Bernardi E et al. A simple ultrasound approach for detection of recurrent proximal-vein thrombosis. *Circulation* 1993;88:1730–5.

8. Froelich JB. Magnetic resonance phlebography. In: Ernst CB, Stanley JC, eds. *Current Therapy In Vascular Surgery, 4th Edn.* St Louis, Missouri: Mosby, 2001:822–4.

9. Begemann PG, Bonacker M, Kemper J et al. Evaluation of the deep venous system in patients with suspected pulmonary embolism with multi-detector CT: a prospective study in comparison to Doppler sonography. *J Comput Assist Tomogr* 2003;27:399–409.

10. Loud PA, Katz DS, Bruce DA et al. Deep venous thrombosis with suspected pulmonary embolism: detection with combined CT venography and pulmonary angiography. *Radiology* 2001;219:498–502.

11. Wells PS, Anderson DR, Rodger M et al. Evaluation of D-dimer in the diagnosis of suspected deep-vein thrombosis. *N Engl J Med* 2003;349:1227–35.

# The role of statins in treating peripheral arterial disease

### Judith G Regensteiner PhD
Department of Medicine, University of Colorado Health Sciences Center, Denver, Colorado, USA

When one is deliberating the use of statins (3-hydroxy-3-methyl-glutaryl CoA reductase inhibitors) in patients with peripheral arterial disease (PAD), two important aspects of treatment should be considered. First, one should consider the use of the statins to treat the increased cardiovascular risk imposed by systemic atherosclerosis. Secondly, the possibility of treating PAD-related symptoms with a statin should be evaluated.

## Treatment of cardiovascular risk associated with atherosclerosis

There is a well-known and substantial overlap between PAD and coronary heart disease (CHD) such that many patients with PAD also have CHD (an estimated 60%).[1] Therefore, patients with PAD are likely to have CHD as well. Despite the overlap of PAD and CHD, however, prospective, randomized trials have not, until recently, shown that treating dyslipidemia decreases cardiovascular morbidity and mortality in patients with PAD. In a meta-analysis of randomized trials in 698 patients with PAD treated with a variety of therapies for lowering lipids, Leng et al. reported a non-significant reduction in mortality and no change in non-fatal cardiovascular events.[2] However, results from the Heart Protection Study (HPS) have recently been published and have unequivocally shown the beneficial effects of statins in patients with PAD.[3] In the HPS, 20 536 adults (aged 40–80 years) from the UK with CHD, other occlusive arterial disease or diabetes were randomly allocated to receive simvastatin, 40 mg daily, or matching placebo in an intention-to-treat design. The patients included 6748 with PAD with and without CHD. Primary outcomes included mortality (for overall analyses) and fatal or non-fatal vascular events (for subcategory analyses). Over a 5-year period, patients with PAD and a history of CHD who received simvastatin had significantly fewer vascular events than those taking placebo (27.6 vs 37.3%). When a subset of 2701 patients with PAD but not CHD was evaluated, a similar level of risk reduction was found (24.7 vs 30.5%). Importantly, whether or not CHD was present, the effect of statins in reducing the risk of vascular events was strikingly significant.[3]

Thus, available data and consensus opinion support the treatment of dyslipidemia in patients with PAD according to the National Cholesterol Education Program (Third Report) guidelines, which recommend maintaining a low-density-lipoprotein cholesterol level below 100 mg/dL.[4]

### Highlights in the role of statins in treating peripheral arterial disease 2003–04

#### WHAT'S IN?
- Consider statin treatment for patients with peripheral artery disease (PAD) because of the high risk of cardiovascular events in this population

#### WHAT'S CONTROVERSIAL?
- The effects of statins on functional capacity in patients with PAD

#### WHAT'S NEEDED?
- More research into the potential functional effects of statins in patients with PAD with claudication and those with 'asymptomatic' disease

## Treatment of PAD-related symptoms

Some data support the use of statins in the treatment of PAD symptoms such as claudication, although more research will be beneficial as results are still not completely clear. The earliest hint that the statins might improve walking ability in patients with claudication was found in the Scandinavian Simvastatin Survival Study. In a subgroup analysis in this study, the reduction in cholesterol level produced by simvastatin was associated with a 38% reduction in the risk of new or worsening symptoms of intermittent claudication.[5]

More recently, administration of atorvastatin has been reported to improve some measures of walking distance and community-based physical activity in patients with intermittent claudication.[6] This study was a randomized, double-blind, parallel-design study in which 354 patients with claudication caused by PAD were studied. Patients were randomized to receive placebo or atorvastatin, 10 mg or 80 mg per day, for 12 months. Mohler et al. reported that maximal walking time after 12 months' treatment with atorvastatin did not change significantly.[6] However, there was improvement in pain-free walking time after 12 months for the 80 mg atorvastatin group compared with the placebo group ($p = 0.025$). In addition, a low-level physical activity questionnaire demonstrated improvement in ambulatory ability for both the 10 mg and the 80 mg atorvastatin groups ($p = 0.011$); however, neither the Walking Impairment Questionnaire nor Short Form 36 Questionnaire showed significant change.[6]

Other studies of statins to treat claudication by improving walking distance are currently being undertaken, and this is an exciting area of inquiry.

Even in patients with PAD who do not have the symptom of claudication (those who have been termed 'asymptomatic' in the past), there is some evidence that statins may have a functional benefit. McDermott et al. reported that patients with PAD who were previously considered asymptomatic in reality have functional limitations.[7] Among 392 patients with an ankle–brachial index (ABI) below 0.90 and 249 patients with an ABI of 0.90–1.50, statin utilization was associated with better functional performance on objective measures of leg functioning than non-utilization.[7]

Although the statin users had several characteristics associated with greater functional impairment than those of non-users, including a higher prevalence of heart disease and stroke and a higher proportion of participants with ABI below 0.90 than non-users, the association between statin use and better functioning remained even after adjustment for potential confounders such as these.[8]

In summary, statins have been shown in a prospective, randomized trial to be effective in preventing vascular events. The effects of statins in improving symptoms affecting functional ability in patients with PAD appear promising, but as yet this remains an area warranting further study.

### References

1. Dormandy J, Heeck L, Vig S. Lower-extremity atherosclerosis as a reflection of a systemic process: implications for concomitant coronary and carotid disease. *Semin Vasc Surg* 1999;12:118–22.

2. Leng GC, Price JF, Jepson RG. Lipid-lowering for lower limb atherosclerosis (Cochrane Review). *Cochrane Database Syst Rev* 2000;(2):CD000123.

3. Heart Protection Study Collaborative Group. MRC/BHF Heart Protection Study of cholesterol lowering with simvastatin in 20,536 high-risk individuals: a randomised placebo-controlled trial. *Lancet* 2002;360:7–22.

4. Executive Summary of The Third Report of The National Cholesterol Education Program (NCEP) Expert Panel on Detection, Evaluation, And Treatment of High Blood Cholesterol In Adults (Adult Treatment Panel III). *JAMA* 2001;285:2486–97.

5. Randomised trial of cholesterol lowering in 4444 patients with coronary heart disease: the Scandinavian Simvastatin Survival Study (4S). *Lancet* 1994;344:1383–9.

6. Mohler ER 3rd, Hiatt WR, Creager MA. Cholesterol reduction with atorvastatin improves walking distance in patients with peripheral arterial disease. *Circulation* 2003;108:1481–6.

7. McDermott MM, Guralnik JM, Greenland P et al. Statin use and leg functioning in patients with and without lower-extremity peripheral arterial disease. *Circulation* 2003;107:757–61.

# Regional anesthesia for vascular surgery

**Farid Moulla** MD and **Avinash Sinha** FRCA

Department of Anaesthesia, Charing Cross Hospital, London, UK

Patients undergoing vascular surgery are at risk for serious perioperative cardiac complications, such as non-fatal myocardial infarction and death. Preoperative screening of vascular patients has revealed that 20% suffer from stress-induced ischemia during dobutamine stress echocardiography.[1] The 1998–2000 surveys from the Vascular Surgical Society of Great Britain and Ireland reported the presence of coexisting cardiac diseases in up to 42% of all cases, with an age-related increase in mortality.[2] Postoperative ischemic events appear to be related to a persistently exaggerated sympathetic response, associated with substantial increases in heart rate throughout perioperative hospitalization.[3]

Major surgery induces profound physiologic changes in the perioperative period, characterized by increased sympathoadrenal neuroendocrine activity and cytokine production.[4] Compared with systemic opioids, epidural anesthesia more effectively attenuates the 'stress response' to surgery, providing better postoperative analgesia and decreased pulmonary complications.[5,6] Perioperative hemodynamic stability is associated with improved peripheral blood flow.[5,7]

The causes of mortality and morbidity following vascular surgery are multifactorial, with anesthetic technique contributing less than surgical factors and postoperative care as a whole. Nevertheless, regional anesthesia, on its own or combined with general anesthesia, has potential benefits, including reduction of intra- and postoperative sympathetic stimulation, with improved postoperative respiratory, cardiovascular, gastrointestinal and coagulation function.[8] Most studies comparing regional anesthesia with general anesthesia in vascular patients have enrolled small cohorts and have failed to show a difference in mortality or morbidity. A meta-analysis published in late 2000, however, showed a reduction in mortality following neuraxial blockade compared with general anesthesia,[9] and, although this study was not specific to vascular surgery, it constituted a landmark for regional anesthesia.

Although evidence for benefits of regional anesthesia on mortality and morbidity for vascular surgery is lacking, enthusiasm for the technique is growing. In the Vascular Surgical Society survey, epidural anesthesia was used in 50% of AAA repairs, 50% of infrainguinal bypass procedures, and 25% of carotid endarterectomies.

### Highlights in regional anesthesia for vascular surgery 2003–04

#### WHAT'S IN?
- Avoiding neuraxial block within 12 hours of the last dose of low-molecular-weight heparin (LMWH)
- Not giving LMWH within 2 hours of an attempted neuraxial block or the removal of an epidural catheter

#### WHAT'S OUT?
- Stopping low-dose (75 mg) aspirin
- Epidurals with peripheral sepsis/gangrene

#### WHAT'S CONTROVERSIAL?
- Delaying surgery or anticoagulation after a bloody tap (epidural needle/catheter)
- Stopping clopidogrel prior to neuraxial block
- Using an anesthetic consent form/fact sheet relating risks and benefits
- Stopping ACE inhibitors for 24 hours perioperatively[25]

More studies are needed, and the results of the general versus local anesthesia (GALA) trial for carotid endarterectomy and the Multicenter Australian Study of Epidural Anesthesia and Analgesia in Major Surgery (MASTER) trial are expected in a couple of years. If they provide strong evidence in favor of regional anesthesia, a change in clinical practice will surely follow. This review discusses evidence for the benefits of regional anesthetic techniques for vascular surgery.

## Abdominal aortic aneurysm (AAA) repair

Ruptured and unruptured AAA repairs are known to have different outcomes.[2] Epidural anesthesia, alone or in combination with general anesthesia, is used in 50% of elective non-ruptured cases, but seldom used in ruptured cases owing to urgency and prevailing fears of clotting abnormalities.

Outcome studies comparing general anesthesia plus epidural anesthesia with general anesthesia alone for major abdominal surgery show transient but quantifiable differences in pain and psychomotor function on emergence from anesthesia.[10] Length of hospital stay and direct medical costs were similar, even when postoperative opiate or epidural patient-controlled analgesia were added to the comparison.[11]

Endovascular aortic aneurysm repair (EVAAR) using a stent graft is an alternative to traditional open repair of AAA. Control of ischemic limb pain due to femoral artery cannulation over a lengthy procedure, rather than control of postoperative surgical pain, is required with this minimally invasive procedure. Monitored sedation with local anesthetic infiltration at the access site is extremely safe and effective; however, continuous epidural or spinal anesthesia can provide more hemodynamic stability and better pain control.[12]

## Infra-inguinal bypass surgery

No distinct advantage has been demonstrated for either regional or general anesthesia in terms of perioperative cardiac morbidity and mortality in peripheral vascular surgery. There is some evidence favoring regional over general anesthesia, however, in optimizing graft patency and reducing the reoperation rate, provided the regional technique is extended to provide postoperative epidural analgesia.[13]

Symptoms of rest pain, gangrene or tissue necrosis may require anticoagulation, which is a relative contraindication to neuraxial block. This is the subject of recent recommendations (see box *What's in and What's out*).[14] Perioperative heparin infusions are not contraindicated in the presence of epidural catheter infusions, but the infusion must be stopped for 4–6 hours, allowing clotting to return to normal, before insertion and removal of the catheter. In the event of a 'bloody tap' with needle or catheter during attempted neuraxial block, there is no consensus as to the correct response. Some clinicians would postpone surgery for 24 hours, others would resite the epidural but wait for 1–2 hours before giving perioperative intravenous heparin.

The risks of neuraxial block in patients with localized peripheral limb sepsis are outweighed by:
- the potential cardiac benefits
- improved peripheral blood flow, coagulation profile and postoperative pain.[6,15,16]

## Carotid endarterectomy

The number of carotid endarterectomy procedures is increasing, because of an aging population and softening of surgical criteria, to include asymptomatic high-grade (> 70%) stenosis.[17] Since the procedure was first introduced in 1954, there has been considerable debate regarding the relative merits of general versus regional anesthesia, but it has recently emerged that regional anesthesia may be associated with a lower morbidity.[18]

Regional anesthesia for carotid surgery offers the advantage of being able to monitor the awake patient's neurologic status continuously during carotid cross-clamping, allowing up to 90% of procedures to be performed without shunting.[19] The ipsilateral cerebral circulation is better preserved, with an increased tolerance of the effects of carotid clamping, under regional anesthesia.[20] In

patients undergoing carotid endarterectomy, greater perioperative hemodynamic stability with regional anesthesia results in:
- fewer major adverse cardiac events
- decreased critical care resource use
- a shortened length of stay.[21]

The perceived advantages of general anesthesia include a reduction in cerebral metabolic oxygen requirement, with greater patient and surgeon comfort. There are no infallible monitors of cerebral ischemia in patients under general anesthesia, however, and the rate of shunting is therefore high, increasing operative time and complication rates.[22] In contrast, regional anesthesia is attractive owing to the resultant reliable clinical monitoring of cerebral perfusion, lower costs and lower mortality and morbidity, thus allowing ambulatory treatment.

The relatively low utilization of regional anesthesia for carotid endarterectomy, compared with infra-inguinal bypass surgery or AAA, relates to apprehensions about learning an unfamiliar technique.[23] Comfortable positioning and conscious sedation with propofol or remifentanil greatly improves patient compliance.[18,24]

### References

1. Poldermans D, Boersma E, Bax JJ et al. The effect of bisoprolol on perioperative mortality and myocardial infarction in high risk patients undergoing vascular surgery. *N Engl J Med* 1999;341:1789–94.

2. Ashley S, Ridler B. *National Vascular Database Report 2002*. The Vascular Surgical Society of Great Britain and Ireland. Dendrite Clinical Systems, 2002.

3. Mangano DT, Layug B, Wallace A, Tateo I. Effect of atenolol on mortality and cardiovascular morbidity after non-cardiac surgery. *N Engl J Med* 1996;335:1713–20.

4. Kehlett H. Multimodal approach to control postoperative pathophysiology and rehabilitation. *Br J Anaesth* 1997;78:606–17.

5. Damask MC, Weissman C, Todd G. General versus epidural anesthesia for femoral-popliteal bypass surgery. *J Clin Anesth* 1990;2:71–5.

6. Ballantyne JC, Carr DB, deFerranti S et al. The comparative effects of postoperative analgesic therapies on pulmonary outcome: cumulative meta-analyses of randomized controlled trials. *Anesth Analg* 1998;86:598–612.

7. Haljamae H, Frid I, Holm J, Akerstrom G. Epidural vs general anaesthesia and leg blood flow in patients with occlusive atherosclerotic disease. *Eur J Vasc Surg* 1988;2:395–400.

8. Liu S Carpenter R, Neal J. Epidural anesthesia and analgesia: their role in postoperative outcome. *Anesthesiology* 1995;82:1474–506.

9. Rodgers A, Walker N, Schug S et al. Reduction of postoperative mortality and morbidity with epidural or spinal anaesthesia: results from overview of randomized trials. *BMJ* 2000;321:1493.

10. Handley GH, Silbert BS, Mooney PH et al. Combined general and epidural anesthesia versus general anesthesia for major abdominal surgery: postanesthesia recovery characteristics. *Reg Anesth* 1997;22:435–41.

11. Norris E, Beattie C, Perler BA et al. Double masked randomized trial comparing alternate combinations of intraoperative anesthesia and postoperative analgesia in abdominal aortic surgery. *Anesthesiology* 2001;95:1054–67.

12. Lippmann M, Lingam K, Rubin S et al. Anesthesia for endovascular repair of abdominal and thoracic aortic aneurysms: a review article. *J Cardiovasc Surg (Torino)* 2003;44:443–51.

13. Breen P, Park KW. General anesthesia versus regional anesthesia. *Int Anesthesiol Clin* 2002;40:61–71.

14. Horlocker TT, Wedel DJ, Benzon H et al. Regional anesthesia in the anticoagulated patient: defining the risks (the second ASRA Consensus Conference on Neuraxial Anesthesia and Anticoagulation). *Reg Anesth Pain Med* 2003;28:172–97.

15. Christopherson R, Glavan NJ, Norris EJ et al. Control of blood pressure and heart rate in patients randomized to epidural or general anesthesia for lower extremity vascular surgery. *J Clin Anesth* 1996;8:578–84.

16. Tuman KJ, McCarthy RJ, March RJ et al. Effects of epidural anesthesia and analgesia on coagulation and outcome after major vascular surgery. *Anesth Analg* 1991;73:696–704.

17. Anon. Randomised trial of endarterectomy for recently symptomatic carotid stenosis: final results of the MRC European Carotid Surgery Trial (ECST). *Lancet* 1998;351:1379–87.

18. McCleary AJ, Maritati G, Gough MJ. Carotid endarterectomy; local or general anaesthesia? *Eur J Vasc Endovasc Surg* 2001;22:1–12.

19. Stoneburner JM, Nishanian GP, Cukingnan RA, Carey JS. Carotid endarterectomy using regional anesthesia: a benchmark for stenting. *Am Surg* 2002;68:1120–3.

20. McCarthy RJ, Nasr MK, McAteer P, Horrocks M. Physiological advantages of cerebral blood flow during carotid endarterectomy under local anaesthesia. A randomized clinical trial. *Eur J Vasc Endovasc Surg* 2002;24:215–21.

21. Sternbach Y, Illig KA, Zhang R et al. Hemodynamic benefits of regional anesthesia for carotid endarterectomy. *J Vasc Surg* 2002;35:333–9.

22. Sundt T, Houser O, Sharbrough F. Carotid endarterectomy: results, complications and monitoring techniques. *Adv Neurol* 1977;16:97–119.

23. Knighton J, Stoneham M. Carotid endarterectomy. A survey of UK anaesthetic practice. *Anaesthesia* 2000;55:481–5.

24. Krenn H, Deusch E, Jellinek H et al. Remifentanil or propofol for sedation during carotid endarterectomy under cervical plexus block. *Br J Anaesth* 2002;89:637–40.

25. Colson P, Ryckwaert F, Coriat P. Renin angiotensin system antagonists and anesthesia. *Anesth Analg* 1999;89:1143.

# Measuring outcomes in vascular surgery

Patrice L Anderson MD, Annetine Gelijns PhD, Alan J Moskowitz MD and K Craig Kent MD

Columbia Weill Cornell Division of Vascular Surgery and International Center for Health Outcomes and Innovation Research, New York Presbyterian Hospital, USA

Measurement of appropriate clinical outcomes is essential in all areas of medicine, because it is only through outcomes assessment that we learn the value of our interventions. Vascular interventions range from medication to complex surgery, and many new 'minimally invasive' techniques compete with existing open surgical procedures. Although these less invasive techniques are often more costly, partly because of the need for re-intervention, they have the advantage of causing less morbidity, mortality and discomfort. These inherent trade-offs lead to questions concerning which approach is best for which type of patient; answering such questions requires consideration of a variety of different outcome measures. Thus, measuring vascular outcomes is a complex task.

Traditional vascular outcomes include mortality, morbidity and patency. Although these endpoints are obviously important and need to be measured, other measures, such as quality of life and cost, are now also important considerations. These outcomes can be evaluated through a variety of study designs, ranging from non-randomized, single-institution case series to multicenter, randomized, controlled clinical trials. Such studies typically involve specialized centers, however, and may not be representative of the outcomes of treatment seen in the community. Assessing the effectiveness of new procedures in everyday practice is best facilitated by the use of large data sets that document a regional or national experience.

As technologic advances in vascular intervention continue, it is imperative that vascular surgeons remain committed to assessing the success of these interventions using a diverse set of outcomes. A broad range of outcome measures is available including clinical effectiveness, quality of life, patient preference and cost, all of which are important and inter-related. A procedure may be clinically effective, but cannot be considered truly successful unless the patient is satisfied and, in the case of limb revascularization, independence is restored. It must also be cost-effective relative to other major medical interventions. Finally, the outcomes of a procedure achieved in single institutional studies should be validated by outcomes derived from large national and regional data sets.

## Data sets

The desire to measure what happens on a large scale, in everyday life, has led to the widespread use of secondary data from large databases, such as those maintained by Medicare. Large data sets fulfill an important role by allowing us to measure broad outcomes in surgical care. Although in recent years there has been an increasing emphasis on randomized trials to discern what does and does not work in surgery, these trials typically include well-defined, largely homogeneous populations, treated at specialized centers with expertise in the disease process being studied. Treatments that produce favorable (efficacious) outcomes in a research setting may not be beneficial (effective) when applied to a different spectrum of patients or treating physicians in everyday practice (Table 1). Medical outcomes in the community hospital may differ tremendously from those published by clinical researchers at academic facilities.[1]

Large databases allow the discovery of benchmarks or standards of care that are applicable at a regional or national level. Such data sets

TABLE 1

**Definitions used in outcome measures**

- Efficacy — The effect of a healthcare intervention on the outcome of care under ideal or experimental conditions
- Effectiveness — The effect of a healthcare intervention on the outcome of care under usual conditions of use

must contain information that characterizes the medical encounter, including information about the patient, the treatment facility, the type of care delivered and the outcome of that care (Table 2).

**Using large databases.** Large databases are inexpensive to use because they are part of an existing infrastructure for data collection. Selection bias inherent in institution-specific studies is minimized, and they provide a comprehensive representation of all patients, physicians, and health-care institutions within a designated area. Large data sets typically represent a vast number of patients; for example, the Medicare file contains 13 million discharges. Large databases can be helpful for studying:
- variations in patient demographics and preoperative comorbidities
- trends over time in procedure use
- efficiency of care, volume–outcome relationships and clinical outcomes.

Large databases also allow examination of the diffusion and

TABLE 2

**The minimum set of variables seen in most discharge databases**

- Date of birth
- Sex
- Place of residence
- Discharge diagnoses or ICD-9 diagnosis codes
- Procedures performed
- Hospital
- Date of admission
- Date of discharge
- Discharge status (death, home, skilled nursing, etc.)
- Patient identifier
- Physician identifier

ICD-9, *International Statistical Classification of Diseases and Related Health Problems*, 9th edn. Geneva: World Health Organization, 1975.

effectiveness of emerging procedures, e.g. endovascular abdominal aortic aneurysm (AAA) repair.[2]

In recent years, the number of vascular interventions that has been evaluated through large data sets has significantly increased. Subjects that have been addressed include:
- mortality after carotid endarterectomy in the elderly[3]
- evolution of mortality for AAA over two decades[4]
- volume-outcome relationships for AAA repair,[5] carotid endarterectomy[6] and other high risk procedures
- regional variation in the use of vascular interventions.[7,8]

The data sets most often used for these evaluations in the USA include the National Hospital Discharge Survey (NHDS), the National Inpatient Survey (NIS), the Medicare database, and a variety of statewide databases.

**Limitations of large databases.** Although large data sets can provide valuable clinical insights, they do have limitations. First, they lack detail in clinical variables. For example, in a statewide data set that we recently analyzed to compare the outcomes of open and endovascular AAA repair, aortic anatomy was not recorded, although it is a factor that must be considered in comparing the outcomes of treatment in non-randomized groups of AAA patients. It is also sometimes difficult to distinguish preoperative comorbidities from postoperative complications. For example, if the therapeutic encounter includes the code for 'stroke', it is unclear whether the patient was admitted with this diagnosis or if it was the consequence of surgical intervention. Furthermore, there is the potential for human error in diagnosis coding, though this appears to be less of an issue when it comes to surgical encounters. In fact, the sensitivity of coding for major vascular procedures is usually over 90%.[9]

## Quality of life
One measure of outcome that is being increasingly used is an assessment of the impact of a disease or its treatment on the life of the patient. Thus, although a femorotibial bypass may be considered successful in a patient who survives the procedure with a patent graft

and a salvaged limb, the same patient may never walk again due to deconditioning or the stress of the procedure. The procedure may have been a success with respect to conventional outcome measures (survival, adverse events and patency), but from the patient's perspective, as measured by quality of life (QoL) assessment tools, the procedure could be characterized as a total failure. Interest in measuring QoL has been increasing since the 1970s.[10] Before 1990, a MEDLINE search with the phrase 'quality of life' yielded about 7500 articles, but in 1990 this number had increased to 34 000.

QoL is an all-inclusive concept that incorporates the ability of the individual to function physically, emotionally and socially.[11] It conveys an overall sense of well-being, including aspects of happiness and satisfaction with life as a whole. More relevant to clinical assessment is health-related QoL, which ignores issues of life satisfaction that are only indirectly related to health. In either case, QoL assessment is broad and subjective, rather than specific and objective.[12] Because many new surgical interventions are now available for chronic disease states such as claudication, QoL and functional status have become increasingly relevant in the evaluation of vascular disease.

Vascular surgeons are increasingly utilizing QoL as an outcome measure for clinical interventions. QoL has been used in the evaluation of treatments for claudication[13] and venous leg ulcers[14] and following femorodistal[15] and other surgical bypasses.[16]

**Categories and instruments.** Tools for measuring QoL fall into two major categories: generic and disease-specific.

*Generic measures* examine general aspects of QoL and are applicable to a wide variety of patients. These techniques are useful when comparing the impact of surgical interventions. An example of a generic QoL measure is the MOS 36-item Short-Form Health Survey (SF-36).[17] This survey has been used to assess QoL in patients living with multiple illnesses and following numerous interventions.

*Disease-specific measures.* In an attempt to evaluate more accurately the impact of an isolated disease or procedure on QoL, researchers have developed specific instruments designed for particular diseases, precise populations or specific interventions. Examples include the Minnesota Living with Heart Failure Questionnaire[18] and the Parkinson's Disease Quality of Life Questionnaire (PDQL).[19] These specific instruments focus on the relevant aspects of the patient population being studied and are more likely to respond to subtle changes in the function of the patients over the period of study.

Over the last few years, many groups have worked on QoL questionnaires specific to vascular surgery, but so far none has been widely accepted.

### Cost-effectiveness

In the mid 1970s, concern began to emerge about the rapidly expanding cost of healthcare, especially with the spread of new technologies such as dialysis for end-stage renal disease and computed tomography.[20] These stimulated interest in assessing the cost-effectiveness of medical practices. The many technological advances in treatment of vascular disease over the last decade have been accompanied by the need to measure their cost-effectiveness. Although many of these technological advances are associated with decreased morbidity and mortality compared with the standard of care, their cost can be substantial.

One outcome used in cost-effectiveness analyses is the cost per quality-adjusted life-year saved. This value is calculated by taking the difference in the costs associated with comparative interventions and dividing it by the difference in health outcomes offered by the procedures, measured in quality-adjusted life years. The cost-effectiveness of comparative procedures can be calculated in the context of a clinical trial, or projections can be made based on probabilistic models (decision-analysis models), which collate data from a variety of studies.

When two treatment approaches are compared for their effect on survival, three possible scenarios may result.
- The procedure of interest can cost less and extend a patient's life. This is a favorable outcome, where the procedure is cost-saving and should clearly be adopted.

## Highlights in **measuring outcomes in vascular surgery** 2003–04

### WHAT'S IN?

- Assessing quality outcomes (beyond clinical outcomes) in vascular surgery by a set of diverse methods
- The use of large databases for the analysis of clinical interventions in the community at large
- Cost-effectiveness analyses

### WHAT'S OUT?

- Relying on only single institutional studies with outcomes of mortality and morbidity as the basis for decision-making in vascular surgery

### WHAT'S NEEDED?

- Continued interest in developing methods to accurately and adequately measure vascular interventional outcomes
- An all-encompassing look at vascular interventional outcomes, including clinical outcomes, quality of life, patient preferences and cost
- Widespread collection of data into large databases that are easily accessible
- The use of patient identifiers in large databases to allow the outcomes of individual patients to be tracked

- The procedure of interest can cost more and reduce life-expectancy. This is an unfavorable outcome and the alternative, rather than the procedure of interest, should be adopted.
- The procedure of interest extends a patient's life but costs more (the most common scenario).

In this last case, it is helpful to compare the cost-effectiveness of the procedure in question to that of other, well accepted interventions, to determine whether it should be adopted. For example, coronary artery bypass grafting for left main disease has a cost-effectiveness ratio of $9500 per quality-adjusted life-year (QALY),[21] whereas dialysis for end-stage renal disease has a much higher cost-effectiveness ratio of $54 400 per QALY,[22] and both of these figures are commonly accepted by 'society' and by payers. The precise value that society is willing to pay for an intervention remains undefined, though most accepted interventions have cost-effectiveness ratios that are less than $100 000 per life-year saved.

Significant progress has been made towards determining the cost-effectiveness of many vascular procedures. Table 3 shows the cost-effectiveness ratios of some of the interventions commonly performed by vascular surgeons.

TABLE 3

**Cost-effectiveness ratios for common vascular surgical procedures**

| Intervention | Cost per life-year or QALY gained |
| --- | --- |
| Coronary artery bypass grafting[21] | $9500 |
| Ultrasonographic surveillance following CEA[23] | $126 950 |
| CEA in symptomatic patients (50-69% stenosis)[24] | $4462 |
| Screening for AAA[25] | $11 215 |
| Endovascular AAA repair[26] | $22 826 |
| Repair of ruptured AAA[27] | $10 754 |

AAA, abdominal aortic aneurysm; CEA, carotid endarterectomy; QALY, quality-adjusted life-year

**References**

1. Roos LL, Roos NP, Fisher ES, Bubolz TA. Strengths and weaknesses of health insurance data systems for assessing outcomes. In: *Modern Methods of Clinical Investigation, Vol 1.* Washington DC: National Academy Press, 1990.

2. Anderson PL, Arons RR, Moskowitz AJ et al. A statewide experience with endovascular abdominal aortic aneurysm repair – rapid diffusion with excellent early results. *J Vasc Surg* 2004;39:10–18.

3. Fisher ES, Malenka DJ, Solomon NA, Bubolz TA, Whaley FS, Wennberg JE. Risk of carotid endarterectomy in the elderly. *Am J Health* 1989;79:1617–20.

4. Heller JA, Weinberg A, Arons R et al. Two decades of abdominal aortic aneurysm repair: have we made any progress? *J Vasc Surg* 2000;32:1091–100.

5. Hannan EL, Kilburn H, O'Donnell JF et al. A longitudinal analysis of the relationship between in-hospital mortality in New York State and the volume of abdominal aortic aneurysm surgeries performed. *Health Serv Res* 1992;27:517–42.

6. Hannan EL, Popp AJ, Tranmer B et al. Relationship between provider volume and mortality for carotid endarterectomies in New York state. *Stroke* 1998;29:2292–7.

7. Wennberg DE, Lucas FL, Birkmeyer JD et al. Variation in carotid endarterectomy mortality in the Medicare population: trial hospitals, volume, and patient characteristics. *JAMA* 1998;279:1278–81.

8. Birkmeyer JD, Sharp SM, Finlayson SR et al. Variation profiles of common surgical procedures. *Surgery* 1998;124:917–23.

9. Fisher ES, Whaley FS, Krushat WM et al. The accuracy of Medicare's hospital claims data: progress has been made, but problems remain. *Am J Public Health* 1992;82:243–8.

10. Gill TM, Feinstein AR. A critical appraisal of the quality of quality-of-life measurements. *JAMA* 1994;272:619–26.

11. Guyatt GH, Feeney DH, Patrick DL. Measuring health-related quality of life. *Ann Intern Med* 1993;118:622–9.

12. Dalkey N, Rourke D. *The Delphi Procedure and Rating Quality of Life Factors. The Quality of Life Concept.* Washington DC: Environmental Protection Agency, 1973:209.

13. Breek JC, Hamming JF, De Vries J et al. The impact of walking impairment, cardiovascular risk factors, and comorbidity on quality of life in patients with intermittent claudication. *J Vasc Surg* 2002;36:94–9.

14. Loftus S. A longitudinal, quality of life study comparing four layer bandaging and superficial venous surgery for the treatment of venous leg ulcers. *J Tissue Viability* 2001;11:14–19.

15. Paaske WP, Laustsen J. Femorodistal bypass grafting: quality of life and socioeconomic aspects. *Eur J Vasc Endovasc Surg* 1995;10:226–30.

16. Seabrook GR, Cambria RA, Freischlag JA, Towne JB. Health-related quality of life and functional outcomes following arterial reconstruction for limb salvage. *Cardiovasc Surg* 1999;7:279–86.

17. Ware JE, Sherbourne CD. The MOS 36-item short-form health survey (SF-36): conceptual framework and item selection. *Med Care* 1992;30:473–83.

18. Rector TS, Kubo SP, Cohn JN. Validity of the Minnesota Living with Heart Failure Questionnaire as a measure of therapeutic response to enalapril or placebo. *Am J Cardiol* 1993;71:1106–7.

19. De Boer AGEM, Wijker W, Speelman JD, De Haes JCJM. Quality of life in patients with Parkinson's disease: development of a questionnaire. *J Neurol Neurosurg Psychiatry* 1996;61:70–4.

20. Rettig RA. Technology assessment – an update. *Invest Radiol* 1991;26:165–73.

21. Weinstein MC, Stason WB. Cost-effectiveness of coronary artery bypass surgery. *Circulation* 1982;66:III56–66.

22. Strange PV, Summer AT. Predicting treatment costs and life expectancy for end-stage renal disease. *N Engl J Med* 1978;298:372–8.

23. Patel ST, Kuntz KM, Kent KC. Is routine duplex ultrasound surveillance after carotid endarterectomy cost-effective? *Surgery* 1998;124:343–51.

24. Patel ST, Haser PB, Korn P et al. Is carotid endarterectomy cost-effective in symptomatic patients with moderate (50–69%) stenosis? *J Vasc Surg* 1999;30:1024–33.

25. Lee TY, Korn P, Heller JA et al. The cost-effectiveness of a 'Quick-Screen' program for abdominal aortic aneurysms. *Surgery* 2002;132:399–407.

26. Patel ST, Haser PB, Bush HL, Kent KC. The cost-effectiveness of endovascular repair versus open surgical repair of abdominal aortic aneurysms: a decision analysis model. *J Vasc Surg* 1999;29:958–72.

27. Patel ST, Korn P, Haser PB et al. The cost-effectiveness of repairing ruptured abdominal aortic aneurysms. *J Vasc Surg* 2000;32:247–57.

# The effect of renal disease on outcomes of vascular surgery

### Peter A McCullough MD MPH FACC FACP FCCP FAHA
Divisions of Cardiology, Nutrition and Preventive Medicine,
William Beaumont Hospital, Royal Oak, Michigan, USA

The current epidemics of obesity and hypertension are driving a secondary epidemic of combined chronic kidney disease (CKD) and cardiovascular disease (CVD).[1,2] CKD is now recognized as an independent risk factor for atherosclerosis.[3] Importantly, it influences outcomes after percutaneous and surgical vascular procedures. As vascular surgeons commonly perform contrast diagnostic and therapeutic procedures in addition to vascular operations, this short review will generalize information from these three interventions.

## CKD and CV risk

CKD is defined through a range of estimated glomerular filtration rate (GFR) values by the US National Kidney Foundation Kidney Disease Outcomes Quality Initiative (KDOQI) (Figure 1). Most studies of CV outcomes have found that a breakpoint for the development of acute renal failure (ARF), restenosis, myocardial infarction, congestive heart failure and CVD death, occurs below an estimated GFR of 60 mL/minute/1.73 m$^2$, which roughly corresponds to a serum creatinine above 1.5 mg/dL in the general population.[4-7] In a recent study of carotid endarterectomy, renal dysfunction, defined as serum creatinine level above 2.0 mg/dL, was an independent predictor of death or stroke at 30 days.[8] Because serum creatinine level is a crude indicator of renal function, and often underestimates renal dysfunction in women and the elderly, it is important to calculate the estimated GFR or creatinine clearance from the serum creatinine value. The Modification of Diet in Renal Disease equation for creatinine clearance is the preferred method, because it does not rely on body weight (Table 1).[2]

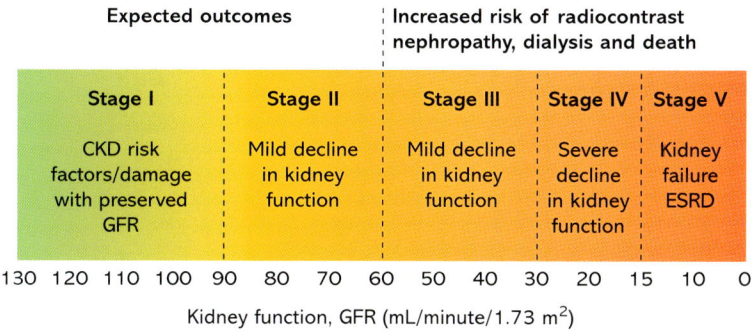

**Figure 1** Classification of the stages of chronic kidney disease (CKD) by the Kidney Disease Outcomes Quality Initiative. Increased rates of adverse events are generally seen below an estimated glomerular filtration rate (GFR) of 60 mL/minute/1.73 m².[2] ESRD, end-stage renal disease.

In a recent study from the US Department of Veterans Affairs' National Surgical Quality Improvement Program concerning lower extremity surgical revascularization, moderate renal insufficiency (estimated GFR 30–59 mL/minute) was associated (within 30 days of lower extremity revascularization) with a significantly increased incidence of:
- postoperative death
- cardiac arrest
- myocardial infarction
- unplanned intubation
- prolonged intubation.[9]

Microalbuminuria at any level of estimated GFR is considered to

---

TABLE 1

**Calculation of creatinine clearance from measured serum creatinine level**

Creatinine clearance = $186.3 \times (\text{serum creatinine}^{-1.154}) \times (\text{age}^{-0.203})$

- × 0.742 for women
- × 1.21 for African Americans

represent CKD and has been thought to occur as the result of hyperfiltration in the kidneys due to diabetes and hypertension-related changes in the glomeruli.[2] Microalbuminuria is now recognized as an independent risk factor for atherosclerosis.[3] A simple definition for microalbuminuria is a random urine albumin/creatinine ratio of 30–300 mg/g. A value above 300 mg/g is usually considered gross proteinuria.

The leading explanations for why CKD (estimated GFR below 60 mL/minute/1.73 m$^2$ or microalbuminuria) is such a potent risk factor for adverse outcomes after vascular procedures include:
- excess comorbidities, such as greater age, diabetes and hypertension
- a pro-atherosclerotic milieu manifested by increased levels of oxidative stress and inflammatory factors.[10]

### Renal artery stenosis as a special case of CKD

The prevalence of renal artery atherosclerosis and, in particular, significant renal artery stenosis in CKD and end-stage renal disease (ESRD) is uncertain. One report estimates that renal artery stenosis (RAS) is present in 2.1% of all new ESRD cases,[11] but as most ESRD cases are not screened for the presence of RAS, this lesion is probably far more common than that. In studies of patients undergoing cardiac catheterizations for a variety of reasons, largely cardiac, the estimated prevalence of stenosis greater than 50–70% in at least one renal artery is 6–8%.[12-14] In an autopsy series of over 2000 patients dying of stroke, at least one renal artery was more than 75% stenosed in 10% of the series.[15]

The management of renal artery stenosis is controversial, and there is a clear need for a randomized trial of angioplasty versus conservative management in patients with unilateral renal artery stenosis.[16] Importantly, if patients with renal artery stenosis undergo contrast procedures, the rates of renal injury appear to be very similar (7–17%) to those expected with cardiac procedures.[17]

## Poor short-term and long-term outcomes

The overall risk of ARF, defined as a transient rise in serum creatinine to more than 25% above the baseline, occurs in about 13% of non-diabetics and 20% of diabetics undergoing contrast procedures (Figure 2).[18] Fortunately, the incidence of ARF leading to dialysis is rare (0.5–2.0%), but when it does occur, it is associated with catastrophic outcomes, including a 36% in-hospital mortality rate and a 2-year survival of only 19%.[18] Transient rises in serum creatinine are directly related to longer stays in intensive care units and hospital wards after bypass surgery.[19]

In patients with ESRD, long-term outcomes after peripheral vascular surgery are poor. In a case-control study, 31 peripheral vascular surgical procedures in 20 patients with ESRD and 64 matched procedures in 57 patients without ESRD were

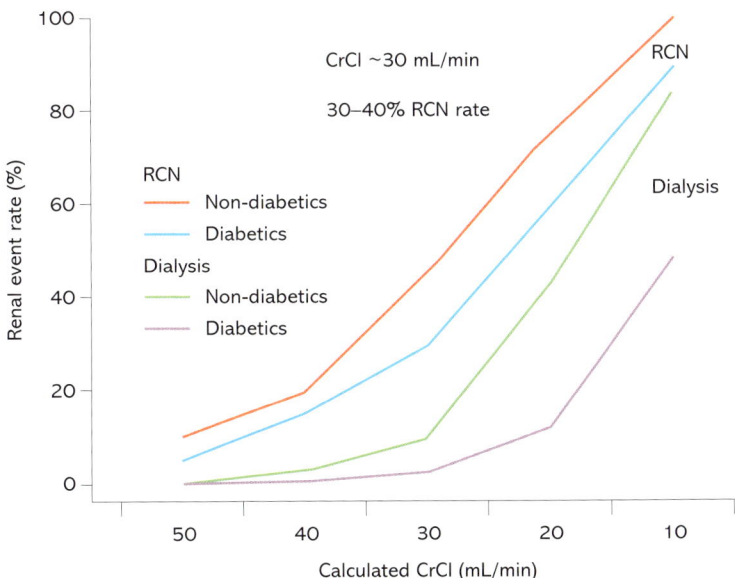

**Figure 2** Validated risk of acute renal failure requiring dialysis after diagnostic angiography and ad hoc angioplasty.[18] This assumes a mean contrast dose of 250 mL for a 72 kg man, mean age 65 years. RCN, radiocontrast nephropathy; CrCl, creatinine clearance.

performed.[20] Median patient survival was significantly shorter in the ESRD group than in the control group (1.7 years versus 5.2 years; $p < 0.001$), as was the time to 50% limb loss (1.2 years versus 5.7 years; $p < 0.001$) and the time to 50% graft patency loss (0.70 years versus 5.5 years; $p < 0.05$). In this study, subjective improvement was also less in patients with ESRD.

### Pathophysiology of renal injury in vascular surgery patients

Three core elements contribute to the pathophysiology of renal injury in vascular procedures (Figure 3):
- direct toxicity of iodinated contrast medium to nephrons
- microshowers of atheroemboli to the kidneys, due to diagnostic catheters, cross-clamping and side-biting of the aorta
- intrarenal vasoconstriction.

Direct toxicity of iodinated contrast medium to nephrons appears to be related to the osmolality of the contrast.

Microshowers of cholesterol emboli are thought to occur in about 50% of percutaneous interventions where a guiding catheter is passed through the aorta.[21] Most of these showers are clinically silent, but in about 1% of high-risk cases, an acute

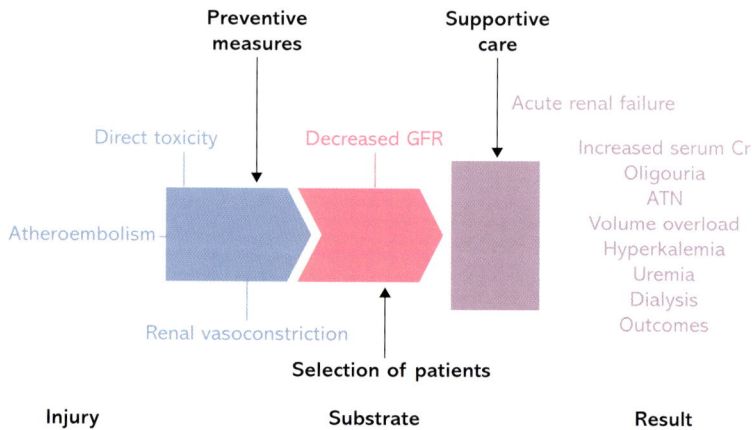

**Figure 3** Model for renal injury occurring with vascular contrast and surgical procedures. GFR, glomerular filtration rate; Cr, creatinine; ATN, acute tubular necrosis.

## Highlights in the effect of renal disease on outcomes of vascular surgery 2003–04

### WHAT'S IN?

- Calculation of estimated glomerular filtration rate (creatinine clearance) from age, gender, creatinine level and race
- Intravenous hydration to a target urine output of 150 mL/hour for at least 6 hours after the procedure
- Iodixanol as the contrast agent of choice
- N-acetylcysteine for renal protection prior to contrast procedures

### WHAT'S OUT?

- Reliance on serum creatinine alone to estimate risk
- 'Renal-dose' dopamine
- Fenoldopam

### WHAT'S CONTROVERSIAL?

- Renal artery angioplasty to preserve renal function in renal artery stenosis
- Use of non-iodinated contrast agents for vascular procedures

### WHAT'S NEEDED?

- A randomized trial of conservative management versus angioplasty for renal artery stenosis
- Large randomized trials of agents to prevent contrast nephropathy and renal injury after vascular surgical procedures

cholesterol–embolic syndrome can develop, manifested by acute renal failure, mesenteric ischemia, decreased microcirculation to the extremities and, in some cases, embolic stroke.

Finally, intrarenal vasoconstriction as a pathologic vascular response to contrast media, and perhaps as an organ response to cholesterol emboli, is a final hypoxic/ischemic injury to the kidney during contrast exposure.[22] Intraoperative hypoxia triggers activation of the renal sympathetic nervous system and results a reduction in renal blood flow.

The most important predictor of acute renal failure is underlying renal dysfunction. The 'remnant nephron' theory postulates that after sufficient chronic kidney damage has occurred and the estimated GFR is reduced to below 60 mL/minute/1.73 m$^2$, the remaining nephrons must pick up the filtration load, have increased oxygen demands, and are more susceptible to ischemic and oxidative injury. Hence, careful selection of patients for procedures is a key element in reducing overall rates of ARF (Figure 2).

### Prevention of acute renal failure

The evidence to date suggests that if a patient can be carried through a vascular procedure without a rise in serum creatinine, a shorter length of stay and improved long-term survival are likely.

Discontinuation of non-steroidal anti-inflammatory agents, aminoglycosides, and ciclosporin before vascular procedures is recommended. These agents all complicate vascular surgery and increase the risk of ARF. For patients with significant CKD (a baseline estimated GFR below 60 mL/minute/1.73 m$^2$), an ARF prevention strategy should be employed, based on:
- hydration
- appropriate choice and quantity of contrast
- pre-, intra-, and post-procedural end-organ protection with pharmacotherapy, to reduce the oxidative stress, which occurs uniquely in CKD patients when exposed to iodinated contrast[18]
- post-procedural monitoring and expectant care.

**Hydration.** When adequate urine flow rates were achieved in a clinical trial setting, there was a 50% reduction in the incidence of ARF.[23] A reasonable approach is intravenous hydration with normal or half-normal saline, starting 3–12 hours before the procedure at a rate of 1–2 mL/kg/hour. In those at risk, at least 300–500 mL of intravenous hydration should be received before contrast is administered. If there are any concerns regarding volume overload or heart failure, right heart catheterization is strongly recommended for management during and after surgery.

A simple intravenous rate to remember from clinical trials of hydration is 150 mL/hour, with a target urine output of 150 mL/hour after the procedure. Importantly, if patients have more than a 150 mL/hour diuresis, the extra losses should be replaced with more intravenous fluid. In general, this strategy calls for hydration orders of normal or half-normal saline at 150 mL/hour for at least 6 hours after the procedure.

**Choice of contrast medium.** The lower the ionic concentration and osmolality of the contrast agent, the less renal toxicity is expected. In a recently completed study, iodixanol (a nonionic, iso-osmolar contrast agent) proved to be superior to iohexol with a lower incidence of ARF observed.[24] Iodixanol has also been demonstrated to be less thrombogenic than other contrast agents, with a 45% reduction in major adverse cardiac events over ioxaglate meglumine.[25] Iodixanol is thus the contrast agent of choice in patients at high renal risk.

In general, it is desirable to limit the amount of contrast medium to below 100 mL for any procedure. If staged procedures are planned and ARF occurs on the first contrast exposure, it is desirable to have more than 10 days between the first and second contrast exposures.

**Pharmacotherapy.** Over 40 randomized trials have tested various strategies in the prevention of ARF[18] and have provided some lessons.
- Diuretics (loop diuretics or mannitol) can worsen ARF if there is inadequate volume replacement for the diuresis that follows.

- Low-dose or 'renal-dose' dopamine cannot be achieved despite its popularity in practice, given the counterbalancing forces of intra-renal vasodilation via the dopamine-1 receptor, and the vasoconstricting forces of the dopamine-2, alpha and beta receptors.
- Various agents, including aminophylline, anaritide, endothelin receptor antagonists and calcium-channel blockers, have not been beneficial.

A large trial of fenoldopam in high-risk patients undergoing cardiac angioplasty showed no benefit for this agent.[26] Of 12 trials of prophylactic N-acetylcysteine (an antioxidant), six trials were positive and six trials were neutral, with an overall edge in favor of the antioxidant (odds ratio for developing ARF, 0.54; 95% confidence interval, 0.29–1.03.[27]

Given the seriousness of ARF as a complication, the relative safety of the strategies used, and the evolution of clinical trials shaping our practice, the combination of hydration, use of iodixanol and N-acetylcysteine is a reasonable three-pronged approach to minimize the incidence of ARF.

**Post-procedural monitoring** is an issue in the modern era of short-stay and outpatient procedures. In general, high-risk patients in hospital should be hydrated starting 12 hours before the procedure and continuing for at least 6 hours afterwards. Serum creatinine should be measured 24 hours after the procedure. For outpatients, particularly those with an estimated GFR below 60 mL/hour, either an overnight stay or discharge to home with 48-hour follow-up and creatinine measurement is advised. It has been shown that those individuals who develop severe ARF have a rise of serum creatinine of more than 0.5 mg/dL in the first 24 hours after the procedure.[28] For those who have not had this degree of creatinine elevation, and have had an otherwise uneventful course, discharge to home may be considered.

**Overall approach.** The items in Table 2 are advised for ARF risk assessment and prevention. It is important that ARF risks are

### TABLE 2
### Checklist for renal risk stratification and prevention for patients at risk undergoing vascular procedures

- Calculate estimated GFR (creatinine clearance): high risk if < 60 mL/minute/1.73 m$^2$
- Check diabetic status: fivefold higher risk if diabetic
- Discuss renal risk in informed consent process
- Discontinue non-steroidal anti-inflammatory drugs and other nephrotoxic drugs
- Nephrology consult for estimated GFR < 15 mL/minute for dialysis planning after PCI
- Hydrate with normal or half-normal saline, 150 mL/hour for 3 hours before and 6 hours after procedure
- Ensure urine flow rate > 150 mL/hour after PCI
- Use iodixanol as preferred contrast agent
- Limit contrast volume to < 100 mL
- *N*-acetylcysteine, 600 mg in 30 mL of ginger ale, orally twice daily for 2 days before and 2 days after PCI

GFR, glomerular filtration rate; PCI, percutaneous coronary intervention

discussed in the consent process. For those with an estimated GFR below 30 mL/minute/1.73 m$^2$, the possibility of dialysis should be mentioned. For those with an estimated GFR below 15 mL/minute/1.73 m$^2$, nephrology consultation is advised, with possible planning for dialysis after the procedure.

## References

1. McCullough PA. Cardiorenal risk: an important clinical intersection. *Rev Cardiovasc Med* 2002;3:71–6.

2. National Kidney Foundation. Clinical practice guidelines for chronic kidney disease: evaluation, classification, and stratification. *Am J Kidney Dis* 2002;2 (suppl 1):S46–75.

3. Sarnak MJ, Levey AS, Schoolwerth AC et al. Kidney disease as a risk factor for development of cardiovascular disease: a statement from the American Heart Association Councils on Kidney in Cardiovascular Disease, High Blood Pressure Research, Clinical Cardiology, and Epidemiology and Prevention. *Circulation* 2003;108:2154–69.

4. McCullough PA, Soman SS, Shah SS et al. Risks associated with renal dysfunction in patients in the coronary care unit. *J Am Coll Cardiol* 2000;36:679–84.

5. Beattie JN, Soman SS, Sandberg KR, Yee J, Borzak S, McCullough PA. Determinants of mortality after myocardial infarction in patients with advanced renal dysfunction. *Am J Kidney Dis* 2001;37:1191–200.

6. Chertow GM, Lazarus JM, Christiansen CL et al. Preoperative renal risk stratification. *Circulation* 1997;95:878–84.

7. Szczech LA, Best PJ, Crowley E et al. Outcomes of patients with chronic renal insufficiency in the bypass angioplasty revascularization investigation. *Circulation* 2002;105:2253–8.

8. Reed AB, Gaccione P, Belkin M et al. Preoperative risk factors for carotid endarterectomy: defining the patient at high risk. *J Vasc Surg* 2003;37:1191–9.

9. O'Hare AM, Feinglass J, Sidawy AN et al. Impact of renal insufficiency on short-term morbidity and mortality after lower extremity revascularization: data from the Department of Veterans Affairs' National Surgical Quality Improvement Program. *J Am Soc Nephrol* 2003; 14:1287–95.

10. McCullough PA. Why is chronic kidney disease the 'spoiler' for cardiovascular outcomes? *J Am Coll Cardiol* 2003;41:725–8.

11. Fatica RA, Port FK, Young EW. Incidence trends and mortality in end-stage renal disease attributed to renovascular disease in the United States. *Am J Kidney Dis* 2001;37:1184–90.

12. Rihal CS, Textor SC, Breen JF et al. Incidental renal artery stenosis among a prospective cohort of hypertensive patients undergoing coronary angiography. *Mayo Clin Proc* 2002;77:309–16.

13. Alhaddad IA, Blum S, Heller EN et al. Renal artery stenosis in minority patients undergoing diagnostic cardiac catheterization: prevalence and risk factors. *J Cardiovasc Pharmacol Ther* 2001;6:147–53.

14. Crowley JJ, Santos RM, Peter RH et al. Progression of renal artery stenosis in patients undergoing cardiac catheterization. *Am Heart J* 1998;136:913–18.

15. Kuroda S, Nishida N, Uzu T et al. Prevalence of renal artery stenosis in autopsy patients with stroke. *Stroke* 2000;31:61–5.

16. Safian RD. Atherosclerotic renal artery stenosis. *Curr Treat Options Cardiovasc Med* 2003;5:91–101.

17. McCullough PA. The use of contrast media in peripheral, combined, and sequential procedures. *Applicat Imaging Cardiac Interv* 2003;Sept:47-52.

18. McCullough PA, Manley HJ. Prediction and prevention of contrast nephropathy. *J Intervent Cardiol* 2001;14:547–58.

19. Mangano CM, Diamondstone LS, Ramsay JG et al. Renal dysfunction after myocardial revascularization: risk factors, adverse outcomes, and hospital resource utilization. *Ann Intern Med* 1998;128:194–203.

20. Reddan DN, Marcus RJ, Owen WF Jr et al. Long-term outcomes of revascularization for peripheral vascular disease in end-stage renal disease patients. *Am J Kidney Dis* 2001;38:57–63.

21. Keeley EC, Grines CL. Scraping of aortic debris by coronary guiding catheters: a prospective evaluation of 1,000 cases. *J Am Coll Cardiol* 1998;32:1861–5.

22. Uder M, Humke U, Pahl M et al. Nonionic contrast media iohexol and iomeprol decrease renal arterial tone: comparative studies on human and porcine isolated vascular segments. *Invest Radiol* 2002;37:440–7.

23. Stevens MA, McCullough PA, Tobin KJ et al. A prospective randomized trial of prevention measures in patients at high risk for contrast nephropathy: results of the P.R.I.N.C.E. study. Prevention of Radiocontrast Induced Nephropathy Clinical Evaluation. *J Am Coll Cardiol* 1999; 33:403–11.

24. Aspelin P, Aubry P, Fransson SG et al. Nephrotoxic effects in high-risk patients undergoing angiography. *N Engl J Med* 2003;348:491–9.

25. Davidson CJ, Laskey WK, Hermiller JB et al. Randomized trial of contrast media utilization in high-risk PTCA: the COURT trial. *Circulation* 2000; 101:2172–7.

26. Stone GW, McCullough PA, Tumlin JA et al. Fenoldopam mesylate for the prevention of contrast-induced nephropathy: a randomized controlled trial. *JAMA* 2003;290:2284–91.

27. Fishbane S, Durham JH, Marzo K, Rudnick M. N-acetylcysteine in the prevention of radio-contrast induced nephropathy. *J Am Soc Nephrol* 2004;15:251–60.

28. Guitterez N, Diaz A, Timmis GC et al. Determinants of serum creatinine trajectory in acute contrast nephropathy. *J Intervent Cardiol* 2002;15:349–54.

# Prediction of outcome from ruptured abdominal aortic aneurysm

Fausto Biancari MD PhD and Tatu Juvonen MD PhD
Division of Cardiothoracic and Vascular Surgery, University of Oulu, Finland

## Improving outcome of abdominal aortic aneurysm rupture

Rupture of an abdominal aortic aneurysm (AAA) puts the patient at an extremely high risk of death, with a mean postoperative mortality rate of about 48% (range 26.9–68.9%).[1,2] These figures, however, do not represent the overall mortality related to ruptured AAA, as many patients either do not reach hospital alive, or die in hospital before surgical repair because they refuse surgery, are moribund, or their operative risk is judged to be prohibitive. Thus, the community mortality rate secondary to ruptured AAA approaches 80%.[3,4] Recent progress in intraoperative and postoperative care has not substantially influenced this mortality rate, though meta-analysis of 171 studies of open repair of ruptured AAA during the last five decades has indicated a 3.5% reduction in mortality per decade. Nevertheless, the community mortality rate related to ruptured AAA is still extremely high. This burden is likely to increase considerably during the next few years, as it has been estimated that the overall incidence of ruptured AAA will increase by 41.3%, from 6.3 to 8.9/100 000 inhabitants, during the next two decades.[4] These data assume even more relevance when it is considered that survivors of open repair of ruptured AAA usually have a good expectancy and quality of life when compared with an age- and sex-adjusted general population.[5]

Ultrasonographic screening for abdominal aortic aneurysm is a logical means to counteract the increasing incidence of ruptured AAA. Recently, the Multicentre Aneurysm Screening Study showed a 53% reduction of aneurysm-related death in men aged 65–74 years who attended the ultrasonographic screening program.[6] After 4 years, the cost-effectiveness of this screening program was at the margin of acceptability, with a probable further improvement of cost-effectiveness over a longer period.[7] The current reduction in health-care resources does not permit extensive ultrasonographic screening programs, however, and improvements in outcomes are only likely to occur if treatment methods and pathways can be improved. Recent small series provided encouragement that endovascular repair of ruptured AAA could significantly lower postoperative mortality compared with that after open repair.[8,9] Larger studies, and possibly randomized trials, are needed to better assess the technical feasibility of this method and its benefits over open repair.

Hospital volume and surgical experience are still the main potentially modifiable variables for better outcome, but the lack of adequate measures to stratify patients' risk prevents any valuable analysis of the results. In fact, individual patient risk is likely to vary significantly from center to center, mainly because of different referral pathways and preoperative selection patterns. Because of these, major efforts have been directed towards identifying risk factors associated with poor outcome after surgery for ruptured AAA, with a view to including them in clinical risk scores. Preoperative definition of the risk of postoperative death after surgery for ruptured AAA is important for preoperative patient selection and to inform the patient's relatives about the operative risk. A few studies have shown that it is possible to stratify patients' risk effectively by simple scoring methods, which would enable a better evaluation of institutional results and planning of better treatment pathways.

## Predictors of immediate postoperative death

**Age** was identified as a significant risk factor for postoperative mortality in four studies that enrolled 3138 patients in total, in which the reported relative risk ranged from 1.9 to 3.1 for every increase of 10 years in age.[2] A recent study summarizing the outcome of surgery for ruptured AAA in 2041 patients found that patients aged over 65 years have a significantly increased risk of in-hospital death (odds ratio 1.98).[10] For those over 70 years of age, the risk of death may be even higher (odds ratio 4.8).[11] Thus, age is one of the most relevant risk factors in patients undergoing surgical repair of ruptured AAA, and advanced age is often considered as a contraindication to surgery.[3,4,12,13]

**Sex.** In a large literature review, Hallin et al.[2] did not identify sex as a significant risk factor for postoperative death after ruptured AAA. Other large studies, however, have suggested that women are at significantly higher risk of dying after surgery for ruptured AAA (odds ratio 1.69–3.0),[10,11] and a disproportionate number of women also die in the community without being referred to hospital for surgical repair.[12,14] It has been suggested that this is related to the greater age of women experiencing rupture of AAA compared with men.[14] It has also been suggested that the association between AAA and severe atherosclerosis may be stronger in women than in men.[12] Indeed, despite the fact that women generally have a better life expectancy, 5-year survival after surgery for ruptured AAA is 62% for women and 71% for men;[12] although this difference is not significant, it points to a more compromised status of women experiencing ruptured AAA than men.

**Renal failure** is one of the most important determinants of immediate and long-term outcome after cardiovascular surgery. In patients undergoing emergency surgery for ruptured AAA, however, the co-existence of renal failure has not uniformly been found to be associated with an increased risk of immediate postoperative death.[2,10,11,15,16] This may be due to the different criteria used to define renal failure, or simply to the overwhelming impact of other risk factors.

**Preoperative shock and cardiac arrest** are by far the most important predictive factors of postoperative death after surgery for ruptured AAA.[2,15–18] These factors are likely to be strongly associated with the presence of free peritoneal rupture, and thus with unstable hemodynamic conditions, which place the patient at risk despite prompt and technically successful repair.

> **Highlights in the prediction of outcome from ruptured abdominal aortic aneurysm 2003–04**
>
> **WHAT'S IN?**
> - Ultrasonographic screening to reduce the death risk of ruptured AAA
>
> **WHAT'S OUT?**
> - Studies focusing on identification of isolated risk factors associated with poor outcome
>
> **WHAT'S NEEDED?**
> - Validation of current stratifying risk scoring methods, and formulation of new ones
> - Comparative evaluation of results for individual hospitals and surgeons, adjusted for patients' operative risk
> - Randomized trials to establish the benefits of endovascular treatment over open repair of ruptured AAA according to patients' operative risk

**Other preoperative risk factors.** In various studies, death after surgery for ruptured AAA has been significantly associated with:
- a history of myocardial infarction[10]
- ischemic changes on ECG[16]
- non-white race[10,11]
- liver disease[10]
- malignancy[10]
- chronic obstructive pulmonary disease[2]
- low hemoglobin concentration[15,16]
- low hematocrit[18]
- low platelet count[19]
- intraperitoneal rupture.[19]

The problem with some of these variables is that they are not easily and reliably obtainable in the emergency setting.

## Risk scoring methods

A few recent studies have evaluated the efficacy of scoring methods to assess the risk of death after surgery for ruptured AAA. Among these, the Acute Physiology and Chronic Health Evaluation (APACHE II)[20] and the Pictures of Standard Syndromes and Undiagnosed Malformations (POSSUM)[13] scales, despite predicting the postoperative outcome, are too complex for routine use in the emergency setting.

**Chen score.** Hsiang et al.[21] showed that Chen et al.'s preoperative scoring method,[17] which includes age, unconsciousness and cardiac arrest, had a positive predictive value of 95% for a calculated preoperative mortality risk of 90%. However, the use of this apparently simple scoring method is made more difficult by its complicated formula for calculation of the individual risk.

**Glasgow aneurysm score.** A simple risk scoring method, the Glasgow aneurysm score, has been developed (Table 1).[22] This was found to predict postoperative death in the 808 patients with ruptured AAA included in the national registry Finnvasc (Finnvasc Study Group, unpublished data). Importantly, when adjusted for hospitals with a volume of more than 50 patients, this scoring system remained an independent predictor of outcome. In this study,

TABLE 1

**Calculating the Glasgow aneurysm score[22]**

- Age in years
- + 17 points for shock
- + 7 points for coronary artery disease
- + 10 points for cerebrovascular disease
- + 14 points for renal disease

however, the Glasgow aneurysm score failed to predict a mortality risk of 100%.

**Hardman Index.** Hardman et al.[16] reported another simple scoring method including:
- age over 76 years
- creatinine level above 0.19 mmol/L
- loss of consciousness after arrival
- hemoglobin concentration below 9 g/dL
- signs of ischemia on ECG.

When three or more of these factors were present, the postoperative mortality rate was 100%. Interestingly, the mortality rate in patients without any of the risk factors was only 16%. Two studies[23,24] also reported a mortality rate of 100% in patients with a Hardman Index score of three or above, whereas in those with a score of zero it was 8% and 18%, respectively. Neary et al.[13] confirmed the validity of the Hardman Index, but their reported mortality rates for scores of three or more or zero were 90% and 35%, respectively.

### References

1. Bown MJ, Sutton AJ, Bell PRF, Sayers RD. A meta-analysis of 50 years of ruptured abdominal aortic aneurysm repair. *Br J Surg* 2002;89:714–30.

2. Hallin A, Bergqvist D, Holmberg L. Literature review of surgical management of abdominal aortic aneurysm. *Eur J Vasc Endovasc Surg* 2001;22:197–204.

3. Adam DJ, Mohan IV, Stuart WP, Bain M, Bradbury AW. Community and hospital outcome from ruptured abdominal aortic aneurysm within the catchment area of a regional vascular surgical service. *J Vasc Surg* 1999;30:922–8.

4. Heikkinen M, Salenius JP, Auvinen O. Ruptured abdominal aortic aneurysm in a well defined geographic area. *J Vasc Surg* 2002;36:291–6.

5. Korhonen SJ, Kantonen I, Pettilä V, Keränen J, Salo JA, Lepäntalo M. Long-term survival and health-related quality of life of patients with ruptured abdominal aortic aneurysm. *Eur J Vasc Endovasc Surg* 2003;25:350–3.

6. Multicentre Aneurysm Screening Study Group. The Multicentre Aneurysm Screening Study (MASS) into the effect of abdominal aortic aneurysm screening on mortality in men: a randomised controlled trial. *Lancet* 2002;360:1531–9.

7. Multicentre Aneurysm Screening Study Group. Multicentre aneurysm screening study (MASS): cost effectiveness analysis of screening for abdominal aortic aneurysms based on four year results from randomised controlled trial. BMJ 2002;325:1135–42.

8. Van Herzeele I, Vermassen F, Duriex C, Randon C, De Roose J. Endovascular repair of aortic rupture. *Eur J Vasc Endovasc Surg* 2003;26:311–16.

9. Peppelenbosch N, Yilmaz N, van Marrewijk C et al. Emergency treatment of acute symptomatic or ruptured abdominal aortic aneurysm. Outcome of a prospective intent-to-treat by EVAR protocol. *Eur J Vasc Endovasc Surg* 2003;26:303–10.

10. Dimick JB, Stanley JC, Axelrod DA et al. Variation in death rate after abdominal aortic aneurysmectomy in the United States. Impact of hospital volume gender, and age. *Ann Surg* 2002;235:579–85.

11. Heller JA, Weinberg A, Arons R et al. Two decades of abdominal aortic aneurysm repair: have we made any progress? *J Vasc Surg* 2000;32:1091–100.

12. Evans SM, Adam DJ, Bradbury AW. The influence of gender on outcome after ruptured abdominal aortic aneurysm. *J Vasc Surg* 2000;32:258–62.

13. Neary WD, Crow P, Foy C et al. Comparison of POSSUM scoring and the Hardman Index in the selection of patients for repair of ruptured abdominal aortic aneurysm. *Br J Surg* 2003;90:421–5.

14. Cassar K, Godden DJ, Duncan JL. Community mortality after ruptured abdominal aortic aneurysm is unrelated to the distance from the surgical centre. *Br J Surg* 2001;88:1341–3.

15. Halpern VJ, Kline RG, D'Angelo AJ, Cohen JR. Factors that affect the survival rate of patients with ruptured abdominal aortic aneurysms. *J Vasc Surg* 1997;26:939–45.

16. Hardman DT, Fisher CM, Patel MI et al. Ruptured abdominal aortic aneurysms: who should be offered surgery? *J Vasc Surg* 1996;23:123–9.

17. Chen JC, Hildebrand HD, Salvian AJ et al. Predictors of death in nonruptured and ruptured abdominal aortic aneurysms. *J Vasc Surg* 1996;24:614–20.

18. Noel AA, Gloviczki P, Cherry KJ Jr et al. Ruptured abdominal aortic aneurysms: the excessive mortality rate of conventional repair. *J Vasc Surg* 2001;34:41–6.

19. Turton EPL, Scott DJA, Delbridge M, Snowden S, Kester RC. Ruptured abdominal aortic aneurysm: a novel method of outcome prediction using neural network technology. *Eur J Vasc Endovasc Surg* 2000;19:184–9.

20. Seiwert AJ, Elmore JR, Youkey JR, Franklin DP. Ruptured abdominal aortic aneurysm repair: the financial analysis. *Am J Surg* 1995;170:91–6.

21. Hsiang YN, Turnbull RG, Nicholls SC et al. Predicting death from ruptured abdominal aortic aneurysms. *Am J Surg* 2001;181:30–5.

22. Samy AK, Murray G, MacBain G. Glasgow aneurysm score. *Cardiovasc Surg* 1994;2:41–4.

23. Boyle JR, Gibbs PJ, King D, Shearman CP, Raptis S, MJ Phillips. Predicting outcome in ruptured abdominal aortic aneurysm: a prospective study of 100 consecutive cases. *Eur J Vasc Endovasc Surg* 2003;26:607–11.

24. Prance SE, Wilson YG, Cosgrove CM, Walker AJ, Wilkins DC, Ashley S. Ruptured abdominal aortic aneurysms: selecting patients for surgery. *Eur J Vasc Endovasc Surg* 1999;17:129–32.

# Where is endovascular management of abdominal aortic aneurysm in 2004?

### Edward Y Woo MD and Jeffrey P Carpenter MD
Division of Vascular Surgery, University of Pennsylvania Medical Center, USA

Endovascular aneurysm repair (EVAR), pioneered by Parodi in the early 1990s, has made significant progress in all aspects. In the early stages of development, stent grafts were used only to repair abdominal aortic aneurysms (AAAs) in patients with comorbidities (e.g. chronic obstructive pulmonary disease or myocardial infarction) significant enough to preclude open repair. With the advent of new technology, the rapid spread of the skill sets needed to place these grafts, and the demonstration that these grafts are not only safe but also durable, EVAR is now being used more commonly in patients who would otherwise undergo an open repair. Nevertheless, EVAR is still in the early stages of development, and long-term follow-up of EVAR patients is essential to assure durable protection from AAA rupture.

## Preoperative evaluation

Conventional open repair remains the standard treatment of AAA. Nevertheless, most patients with AAA are elderly with multiple co-morbidities, making EVAR an attractive alternative to conventional surgery. The indications for repair with respect to AAA size, growth rate and symptoms remain the same for open and endovascular repair, and the threshold for intervention has not been altered by the advent of minimally invasive therapy.

Although tremendous strides have been made in the development of stent grafts, EVAR is limited by aortic anatomy. Detailed and accurate imaging combined with careful preoperative planning are essential for the intraoperative success of EVAR. Traditionally, AAAs were sized by computed tomography (CT) and contrast angiography for diameter and length, respectively. Although this provides accurate measurements, angiography necessitates an additional procedure. All the necessary information can now be generated from special CT protocols, which involve fine-cut scans (≤ 3 mm) from the diaphragm to the femoral vessels with and without intravenous contrast (no oral contrast is used). Three-dimensional images can be generated from these scans, which provide accurate diameter and length measurement data (Figure 1).[1]

Preoperative planning is the key to successful EVAR. Poor planning leads to an increased rate of endoleaks, complications, open conversion and failure of endograft placement. Achieving an adequate proximal and distal seal requires sufficient length of suitable arterial attachment zones. To obtain this, length and diameter are clearly important, but the angulation, the presence of thrombus or calcification, and the shape of the neck are also important.[2] For example, circumferential thrombus would probably prevent an adequate seal between the graft and the aortic wall, predisposing to an endoleak. Other factors important to graft placement include:

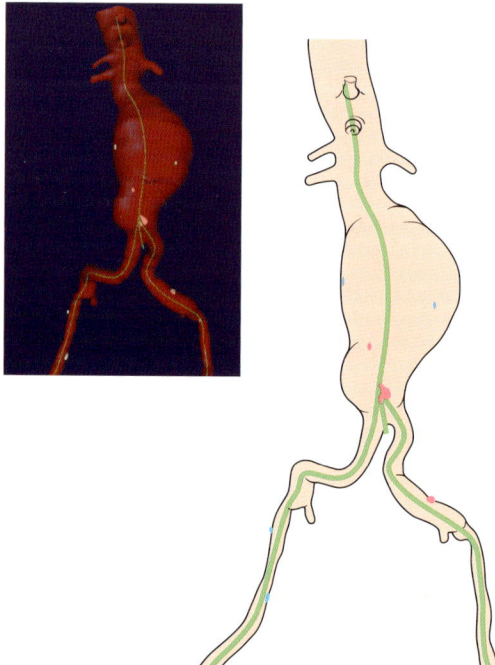

Figure 1 Three-dimensional reconstruction of an AAA showing center-line measurement (green line) and original generated image (inset).

- the presence of accessory vessels that might be covered by the graft
- a narrow aortic bifurcation
- tortuous iliac vessels
- small femoral vessels.

Narrow bifurcations can be treated with aorto-uni-iliac grafts, coil embolization of the contralateral common iliac artery, and subsequent femorofemoral bypass with excellent durability.[3,4] Tortuous iliac vessels and small femoral arteries were traditionally circumvented with an iliac conduit.[5] With low-profile and increasingly flexible devices, conduits are now seldom necessary.

## Graft choice

Since the first stent graft placement in the early 1990s, many types of grafts have undergone clinical trials. The first graft to attain US Food and Drug Administration (FDA) approval was the Ancure graft (Guidant, Menlo Park, CA), which was an unsupported, unibody graft. This device was recently removed from the market, but three other grafts are currently approved by the FDA:

- AneuRx (Medtronic, Minneapolis, Minnesota)
- Excluder (W.L. Gore and Associates, Flagstaff, Arizona)
- Zenith (Cook, Bloomington, Indiana).

All are based on a self-expanding, supported, modular system. Many other grafts are currently in various stages of development.

Of the FDA-approved devices, the Zenith allows for treatment of a larger neck, the Excluder has the smallest delivery system, and the AneuRx has the most long-term data. Unique to the Zenith graft is a transrenal fixation system. Although this does not act as a seal zone, it does provide additional proximal fixation. Furthermore, it does not appear to adversely affect renal function.[6]

Results from two large series of patients were recently published comparing the Ancure, AneuRx, Excluder, Talent (Medtronic) and Zenith devices.[7,8] Risk of rupture and aneurysm-related death among all devices was extremely low. Although there was an overall 15% requirement for secondary procedures, this also did not differ among devices. However, the incidence of endoleak, specifically type II, was greatest with the Excluder. Furthermore, sac shrinkage of more than 5 mm occurred least often with the Excluder (15% at 12 months), though the significance of this is unclear.

As technology advances, newer devices will continually be developed. Each generation of device will address limitations of its predecessors, and will help to broaden the applicability of stent grafts. Different devices will offer different advantages and disadvantages, so the choice must be tailored to each individual patient. Finally, familiarity and confidence with each device will allow the physician the greatest repertoire for treating AAAs.

## Endoleaks

**Classification.** Endoleaks are categorized by type.
- Type I endoleaks involve an inadequate proximal or distal seal.
- Type II endoleaks result from back-flow from collaterals, e.g. lumbar arterial branches or the inferior mesenteric artery.
- Type III endoleaks arise from defects in the fabric or modular component junctional seal zones.
- Type IV endoleaks are secondary to the porous nature of graft fabrics and resolve after reversal of the anticoagulation employed for the EVAR procedure.

**Treatment** and timing of treatment of endoleaks varies between the different types. After insertion of the graft, any type I or III endoleaks detected on the completion angiogram need to be corrected before surgery is concluded. Conversely, type II and IV leaks should simply be observed. Follow-up entails plain radiographs to assess the integrity and position of the stents, and CT angiography at 1 month, 6 months, 1 year, and annually thereafter. Intervention for type II endoleaks is usually reserved for cases of sac enlargement, or a lack of evidence of sac shrinkage after 1 year in the face of a persistent type II endoleak.

Detection and treatment of endoleaks is still in evolution. Endoleaks are mainly first identified by CT angiography, usually by the presence of contrast within the sac. Further definition of the

> **Highlights in endovascular management of abdominal aortic anenysm 2003–04**
>
> **WHAT'S IN?**
> - Three FDA-approved devices: AneuRx, Excluder, Zenith
> - Three-dimensional reconstructions of CT angiography used for sizing
> - New ways of detecting and characterizing endoleaks
> - Development of fenestrated grafts to bridge the visceral and renal components
>
> **WHAT'S OUT?**
> - The Ancure device (removed from the market)
> - Preprocedural angiography for measurements

leak is performed by contrast angiography. Selective injection of the superior mesenteric artery can be helpful in diagnosis of inferior mesenteric endoleaks, and selective hypogastric artery injection can reveal iliolumbar leaks. Duplex scanning for an endoleak is an alternative, but in most hands is less reliable than CT angiography.[9] Much interest has developed in pressure sensors that can be affixed to the graft material and then transfer measurements of sac pressure non-invasively. Elevated sac pressures are hypothesized to correlate with either an endoleak or endotension, and possibly with subsequent rupture. Measurements of isolated areas within the sac, however, may not be reliable as a predictor of rupture, as the pressures may vary within the sac.[10] However, monitoring of the entire sac might be a non-invasive method of predicting which patients need intervention.

Treatment of endoleaks is tailored to the type of leak. Type I or III endoleaks can usually be treated with the addition of new graft material to improve a seal, cover a junction, or cover a defect.

Uncovered stents can sometimes be used to improve a proximal or distal seal zone by increasing the radial force. *n*-Butyl cyanoacrylate adhesive has been used successfully for the treatment of type I endoleaks.[11] Type II endoleaks can be treated by transarterial superselective cannulation of the offending vessel with subsequent coil embolization. Alternatively, direct coil embolization by a translumbar approach may offer better results.[12] Direct thrombin injection of the sac has also been reported.[13] Ultimately, open aneurysm repair and explanting of the stent graft can be performed if other measures have failed.

### References

1. Wyers MC, Fillinger MF, Schermerhorn ML et al. Endovascular repair of abdominal aortic aneurysm without preoperative arteriography. *J Vasc Surg* 2003;38:730–8.

2. Dillavou ED, Muluk SC, Rhee RY et al. Does hostile neck anatomy preclude successful endovascular aortic aneurysm repair? *J Vasc Surg* 2003; 38:657–63.

3. Yilmaz LP, Abraham CZ, Reilly LM et al. Is cross-femoral bypass grafting a disadvantage of aortomonoiliac endovascular aortic aneurysm repair? *J Vasc Surg* 2003;38:753–7.

4. Hinchliffe RJ, Alric P, Wenham PW, Hopkinson BR. Durability of femorofemoral bypass grafting after aortouniiliac endovascular aneurysm repair. *J Vasc Surg* 2003;38:498–503.

5. Abu-Ghaida AM, Clair DG, Greenberg RK et al. Broadening the applicability of endovascular aneurysm repair: the use of iliac conduits. *J Vasc Surg* 2002; 36:111–17.

6. Cayne NS, Rhee SJ, Veith FJ et al. Does transrenal fixation of aortic endografts impair renal function? *J Vasc Surg* 2003; 38:639–44.

7. Sampram ES, Karafa MT, Mascha EJ et al. Nature, frequency, and predictors of secondary procedures after endovascular repair of abdominal aortic aneurysm. *J Vasc Surg* 2003;37:930–7.

8. Ouriel K, Clair DG, Greenberg RK et al. Endovascular repair of abdominal aortic aneurysms: device-specific outcome. *J Vasc Surg* 2003; 37:991–8.

9. Raman KG, Missig-Carroll N, Richardson T et al. Color-flow duplex ultrasound scan versus computed tomographic scan in the surveillance of endovascular aneurysm repair. *J Vasc Surg* 2003;38:645–51.

10. Vallabhaneni SR, Gilling-Smith GL, Brennan JA et al. Can intrasac pressure monitoring reliably predict failure of endovascular aneurysm repair? *J Endovasc Ther* 2003;10:524–30.

11. Maldonado TS, Rosen RJ, Rockman CB et al. Initial successful management of type I endoleak after endovascular aortic aneurysm repair with *n*-butyl cyanoacrylate adhesive. *J Vasc Surg* 2003;38:664–70.

12. Baum RA, Carpenter JP, Golden MA et al. Treatment of type 2 endoleaks after endovascular repair of abdominal aortic aneurysms: comparison of transarterial and translumbar techniques. *J Vasc Surg* 2002;35:23–9.

13. Ellis PK, Kennedy PT, Collins AJ, Blair PH. The use of direct thrombin injection to treat a type II endoleak following endovascular repair of abdominal aortic aneurysm. *Cardiovasc Intervent Radiol* 2003; Nov 21.

# Complications of arteriovenous fistula

**Michael Walter** MD **and Ulrich Boesger** MD
Department of Vascular and Thoracic Surgery, St. Johannes-Hospital,
Duisburg, Germany

Complications following the formation of an arteriovenous fistula are relatively common, and as a result nearly 50% of patients are faced with the necessity of secondary corrective operations during the course of their hemodialysis.[1-4] This is partly due to the fact that the formation of an arteriovenous fistula creates non-physiologic conditions by its very nature, and partly due to the considerable mechanical alteration of the arteriovenous fistula during the course of chronic hemodialysis. The risk of complications following arteriovenous fistula formation can be minimized by obtaining an accurate preoperative diagnosis and by conducting a careful evaluation of the arterial and venous vascular status. If the clinical examination alone proves insufficient, then the entire spectrum of functional and imaging methods (Doppler and duplex ultrasonography, angiography, venography and MRI) can be implemented before surgery.[5,6]

This review discusses only problems related to native fistulas, as problems with alloplastic arteriovenous shunts are of a similar nature and the therapeutic strategies for correction of both types are similar. The review is written from the perspective of a high-volume center, performing about 400 arteriovenous fistula operations per year. The cited literature does not represent the authors' opinion in all cases.

Complications are best categorized by their chronologic progression (early, medium-term and longer term), and the spectrum of therapeutic methods varies accordingly.[7]

## Early complications

Early complications include:
- thrombosis

- postoperative hemorrhage
- damage to the nervous system
- steal syndrome
- early infections.[7]

**Thrombosis.** Early shunt thrombosis is of particular significance. The most common causes of early thrombosis are misjudgment of the arterial and venous status (inadequate inflow/outflow) and technical faults. Only very occasionally does previously unrecognized hypercoagulability play a part in development of early shunt failure.

*Errors of indication.* If the arterial and venous status is misjudged, it is inherently impossible to establish a satisfactory shunt situation. A more central shunt position will have to be selected, e.g. by abandoning a Cimino fistula in the region of the wrist in favor of an arteriovenous connection in the crook of the elbow. In some cases it may be necessary to switch to another extremity, e.g. the contralateral arm, while in others a prior vascular reconstruction, e.g. dilatation of the subclavian artery or reconstruction of venous outflow discharge conditions in the region of the large veins, can prove advantageous and lead to satisfactory fistula function.[8]

*Technical errors* are the most common cause of an early thrombosis of an arteriovenous shunt.
- If venous torsion occurs, it is necessary to renew the anastomosis or perform a detorsion with end-to-end venovenostomy.
- Bending of the fistula vein can be corrected by further mobilizing the vein in a central direction.

Other technical faults are related to the anastomotic configuration. In principle, we recommend an arteriotomy of at least 0.5 cm in length with a corresponding vein size. An adequately sized anastomosis also serves to prevent subsequent complications, such as neointimal hyperplasia, which can lead to a constriction of the anastomosis. If problems with the configuration of the anastomosis result in early thrombosis, reconstruction can be attempted. In the event of longer term shunt thrombosis, however, it is more often

> **Highlights in complications of arteriovenous fistula 2003–04**
>
> **WHAT'S IN?**
> - Native arteriovenous fistula
> - Determination of exact preoperative arterial and venous status
> - Fistula follow-up examination (flow, dialysis pressure) before patient experiences occlusion of the fistula
> - Interventional correction of poor inflow/outflow for stenoses of large vessels
> - Large anastomosis
>
> **WHAT'S OUT?**
> - Occlusion of fistula due to overlooked prior dysfunction
> - Interventional treatment of anastomotic stenosis
>
> **WHAT'S CONTROVERSIAL?**
> - When to apply a reserve procedure

necessary to undertake proximal relocation of the anastomosis after appropriate diagnostic investigations.

If inflow/outflow are uninterrupted, and shunt failure cannot be ascribed to technical faults, then hypercoagulability may be the cause. In such cases, it is advisable to conduct a comprehensive assessment of coagulation status, particularly bearing in mind factor V mutations, lack of protein C and protein S, and thrombocyte disorders, e.g. sticky platelet syndrome.

**Postoperative hemorrhage.** Treatment of postsurgical bleeding should follow general surgical principles.

**Damage to the nervous system** only very occasionally requires surgical re-intervention. If essential motor nerve fibers are affected, the appropriate neurosurgical intervention should follow.

**Steal syndrome,** which can lead to a critical lack of circulation in the hand, may occur as both an early and a medium-term complication.[9] The most common cause of cubital fistula is drainage via the vena cephalica and the vena basilica. It is generally sufficient in these cases to ligate the vena basilica. In individual cases, an exact diagnosis may be necessary in order to facilitate specific reduction of the venous cross-section by constriction of the anastomosis or by banding the discharging vein. In some cases it may prove necessary to abandon the shunt altogether. Shunt reduction can also be achieved by means of a venovenous PTFE interposition, which increases the drainage resistance in the shunt.

## Medium-term complications

Medium-term complications include poor shunt development, steal syndrome and localized or generalized lymphatic edema.[4]

**Poor shunt development.** Unsatisfactory development of a shunt after an initially successful installation, so that it proves unsuitable for dialysis purposes despite clinically sufficient shunt function, has predominantly the same causes as early shunt thrombosis:
- inadequate arterial inflow
- disregarded venous drainage problems
- an inadequate cross-section of the anastomosis.

In such cases, specific additional diagnostic measures, if necessary with angiography or venography, are required. The subsequent corrective measures are dependent on the causes identified, but, in general, it will be necessary to correct the anastomosis, to relocate the shunt (in a minority of cases to the other arm) or to correct arterial and venous stenoses.

**Steal syndrome.** The development of a medium-term steal syndrome following an initially successful shunt development has the same causes as described for the short-term steal syndrome. The therapeutic recommendations also do not differ in principle.

**Lymphatic edema.** Medium-term complications in connection with the lymphatic system are not a common occurrence. Localized lymphatic edema can occur in the region of the surgical incision, but is generally benign and does not require specific treatment. Generalized lymphatic edema often necessitates abandoning the arteriovenous fistula so that adequate external compression can be applied.

**Retrograde venous arterialization.** Generalized lymphatic edema must be distinguished from retrograde venous arterialization, that is, retrograde filling of the fistula vein exits to discharging secondary side branches. This syndrome manifests itself clinically as substantial swelling of the distal veins or even total venous congestion causing substantial impairment of manual functions. The pathophysiologic mechanism is similar to that of chronic venous insufficiency of the lower extremities. In the early stages of retrograde venous arterialization, ligature of the respective side-branches almost always achieves rapid and drastic improvement.

## Long-term complications

The most common long-term complications are stenosis of the discharging veins and congestion of the arteriovenous fistula. In addition, venous aneurysms can develop after years of dialysis punctures (Figure 1).[2,10] Infections may occur, but are more common with alloplastic shunts than native arteriovenous fistulas.

**Stenosis.** Although stenosis of the anastomosis itself can occur, under high-flow conditions neointimal hyperplasia in the discharging vein may occur by a similar pathological mechanism as is found in peripheral bypass anastomoses. In such cases, extreme hardening of the venous walls often precludes the type of corrective interventions that are employed in peripheral bypass surgery. Local desobliteration, e.g. thromboendarterectomy, is also not usually

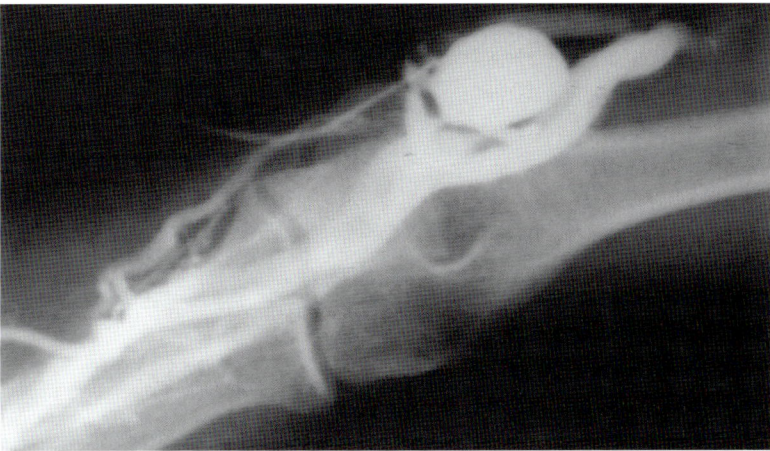

**Figure 1** Large venous aneurysm near the anastomosis of a Cimino fistula at the wrist. It was treated by dissection of the multiple arteriovenous and venovenous fistulas and end-to-end venovenostomy, with good postoperative fistula function.

possible, and more often than not a new shunt is required. The further proximal a stenosis is located from a venous anastomosis, the easier it is to undertake endovascular corrections. Long venous stenoses, e.g. along the course of the vena cephalica following the puncture of a Cimino fistula in the wrist, may be treated successfully with thromboendarterectomy with Rififi maneuver.

In general, for late venous stenoses, the more centrally located the vein is, the more successful the treatment by interventional procedures, for example angioplasty of the axillaris vein.

**Congestion or occlusion** of a native arteriovenous fistula is not usually correctable by simple thrombectomy, as several causes may contribute to the shunt failure. In many of these cases, a new shunt is required, which in some patients with worn-out veins may need to be a synthetic shunt.

**Infections.** Complications caused by infections are rare, but can potentially lead to lethal bleeding through erosion of the vessel wall. In most cases, local debridement will produce secondary healing, but will not avoid the necessity of abandoning the shunt.

## Reserve procedures

Despite the frequency of complications of shunt surgery in preparation for hemodialysis, there are normally many corrective surgical procedures available. If it is no longer possible to construct an arteriovenous fistula (even an alloplastic shunt), as often occurs with younger patients who have undergone many years of dialysis, then the so-called reserve procedures, such as atrial implants (e.g. Demers catheter) or peritoneal dialysis, should not be disregarded.[3] Figure 2 presents a therapeutic algorithm that encompasses all these options.

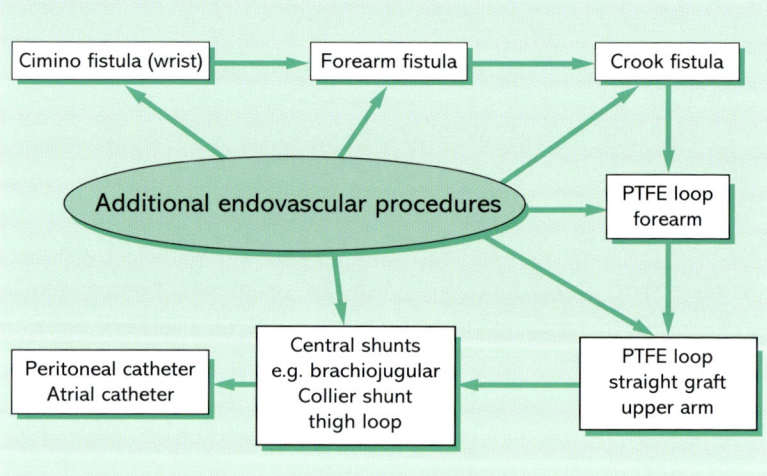

Figure 2 Management of arteriovenous fistula failure.

### References

1. Akoh JA, Dutta S. Autogenous arteriovenous fistulas for haemodialysis: a review. *Niger Postgrad Med J* 2003;10:125–30.

2. Sulkowski U, Schulte H. Arguments in favour of a homologous concept for hemodialysis access procedures. Feasibility and results. *Eur J Vasc Endovasc Surg* 2003;26:96–9.

3. Elseviers MM, Van Waeleghem JP, European Dialysis and Transplant Nurses Associations/European Renal Care Association. Identifying vascular access complications among ESRD patients in Europe. A prospective Multicenter study. *Nephrol News Issues* 2003;17:61–4, 66–8, 99.

4. Grapsa EJ, Paraskevopoulos AP, Moutafis SP et al. Complications of vascular access in hemodialysis (HD) – aged vs adult patients. *Geriatr Nephrol Urol* 1998; 8:21–4.

5. Parmley MC, Broughan TA, Jennings WC. Vascular ultrasonography prior to dialysis access surgery. *Am J Surg* 2002;184:568–71; discussion 572.

6. Konner K, Hulbert-Shearon TE, Roys EC, Port FK. Tailoring the initial vascular access for dialysis patients. *Kidney Int* 2002;62:329–38.

7. Beathard GA, Arnold P, Jackson J et al. Aggressive treatment of early fistula failure. *Kidney Int* 2003;64:1487–94.

8. Tonelli M, Hirsch D, Clark TW et al. Access flow monitoring of patients with native vessel arteriovenous fistulae and previous angioplasty. *J Am Soc Nephrol* 2002;13:2969–73.

9. Meyer F, Muller JS, Grote R et al. [Fistula banding – success-promoting approach in peripheral steal syndrome.] *Zentralbl Chir* 2002;27:685–8.

10. Najibi S, Bush RL, Terramani TT et al. Covered stent exclusion of dialysis access pseudoaneurysms. *J Surg Re*s 2002;106:15–19.

# Blood conservation in thoracic aortic surgery with total cardiopulmonary bypass

### Etsuro Suenaga MD
Department of Cardiovascular Surgery, Nagasaki Kouseikai Hospital, Nagasaki, Japan

Advances in medical technology have led to improvements and refinements in cardiovascular surgery. In turn, these have resulted in greatly improved success rates. It is now possible to undertake ordinary cardiac surgery, such as coronary artery bypass grafting or valve surgery, without using blood transfusion. However, thoracic aortic surgery is one of the most invasive procedures in cardiac surgery, because of prolonged cardiopulmonary bypass time associated with deep hypothermic circulatory arrest, and large blood transfusions are usually unavoidable. A large amount of homologous transfusion still has significant risks, such as viral infection, graft versus host disease, hemolytic reaction and systemic inflammatory response syndrome, which can lead to multiple organ failure.[1,2] Prolonged extracorporeal circulation times too cause a systemic inflammatory response, which may lead to multiple organ dysfunctions.[3,4] Moreover, deep hypothermia increases the risk of hemorrhage.[5] Thoracic aortic surgery is one area in which our methods are changing.

This chapter describes my group's retrospective investigation of blood conservation in thoracic aortic surgery using total coronary pulmonary bypass (CPB).

From December 1997 to May 2000, 59 consecutive patients who underwent thoracic aortic graft replacement with total CPB were studied. Of these, 23 patients had ascending aortic replacement, 21 total aortic arch replacement and 10 aortic root reconstruction, and 5 underwent concomitant aortic root reconstruction and total aortic arch replacement. In 32 cases, surgery was elective; 27 patients had emergency operations. The average age was 67.3 ± 10.8 years, and the male-to-female ratio was 36:23.

### TABLE 1
**Preoperative patient characteristics**

|  | N group (n = 40) | T group (n = 19) | p value |
|---|---|---|---|
| Elective:emergency | 27:13 | 5:14 | < 0.01 |
| Men:women | 30:10 | 6:13 | < 0.01 |
| Age (years) | 66 ± 9.9 | 70 ± 12 | NS |
| Body weight (kg) | 61 ± 10 | 50 ± 10 | NS |
| Hematocrit (%) | 39.0 ± 4.1 | 32.1 ± 5.1 | < 0.01 |
| Platelets (× 10⁴/mL) | 20.0 ± 5.5 | 17.4 ± 6.9 | NS |
| Blood transfusion index | 2320 ± 784 | 1445 ± 706 | < 0.001 |

N group, patients not receiving blood transfusion; T group, patients receiving blood transfusion; NS, not significant

Patient characteristics are shown in Table 1. The patients were divided into two groups: those who underwent graft replacement without blood transfusion (the N group), and those who needed blood transfusion (the T group). Each group was compared for age, sex, emergency status, hematocrit, CPB time, blood transfusion index and operative mortality. Additionally, we investigated the significance of a blood transfusion index above 2000.

### Preoperative autologous blood collection

Preoperative blood collection has been introduced widely in cardiovascular surgery.[6-9] Human recombinant erythropoietin (rHuEPO) combined with iron sulfate is more effective than either agent singly.[10-13]

For each patient having elective surgery in our study, a total of 1200 mL of autologous blood was collected preoperatively. For 3 weeks, 400 mL of whole blood was collected once a week, and patients received Ringer lactate solution at the same time. Recombinant HuEPO, 24 000 units, was injected under the skin, and patients also received iron sulfate orally, 100 mg daily, just before surgery.

**Biocompatibility of the cardiopulmonary bypass system**
To reduce the effects of CPB, a heparin-coated system that included a membrane oxygenator was used. It appears that this type of system might reduce the requirement for autologous blood transfusion.[14–16] In addition, it is interesting to note that, in a canine model, the use of a centrifugal pump and a lower priming volume in the CPB system led not only to a reduction in the requirement for transfused blood but also to suppression of complement activation.[17]

Heparin, 250 IU/kg, was prescribed for the patient, and the activated clotting time was maintained at 300 seconds or greater. The priming volume of the CPB system was also standardized (1100 mL) for biocompatibility. In the operating theater, a cell saver was used for bleeding and the extracorporeal ultrafiltration method was used for hemodilution during CPB.[18] A total of 2 million units of aprotinin was used, 1 million units for the patient and 1 million units for the CPB circuit.[19–22]

The hematocrit criteria for autologous blood transfusion were:
- hematocrit below 18% during CPB time
- hematocrit below 25% in the intensive care unit.

**Blood transfusion index**
The blood transfusion index (preoperative hematocrit × body weight) is a very useful tool for estimating the amount of autologous blood that will be required.

**Results**
Of the 59 consecutive patients who underwent thoracic aortic graft replacement with total CPB, 2 patients had to be returned to the operating theater for postoperative bleeding, and 7 patients died within 30 days of the operation. Of these, five had emergency surgery and the other two had had elective procedures, making the operative mortality rates 6.2% and 18.5% for the elective and emergency procedures, respectively. An autologous blood transfusion was not required by 67.8% of patients: 48.1% (13/27) of those having emergency surgery did not require a transfusion,

> **Highlights in blood conservation in thoracic aortic surgery 2003–04**
>
> **WHAT'S IN?**
> - Preoperative blood donation using rHuEPO and iron sulfate
> - Heparin-coated lower priming volume in the cardiopulmonary bypass system
> - Intraoperative blood salvage
> - Pharmacological therapy
> - Blood transfusion index
>
> **WHAT'S OUT?**
> - Perioperative bleeding due to inadequate procedure
> - Wastage of large amounts of blood products

and nor did 84.4% (27/32) of those having an elective procedure. When analyzed by sex, freedom from blood transfusion was significantly lower in women than in men, 43.3% (10/23) compared with 83.3% (30/36), respectively. The mean quantity of homologous blood required was 5.6 U ± 3.2 U.

The average preoperative hematocrit value and body weight were significantly higher in the N group than in the T group, resulting in a higher average blood transfusion index (Table 1). There were no significant differences in terms of CPB time, cardiac arrest time, circulatory arrest time and lowest rectal temperature. There was significantly more postoperative (12 hours) bleeding in the T group than in the N group (Table 2). The operative mortality rate was also significantly higher in the T group than in the N group, 26.3% (5/19) and 5.0% (2/40), respectively (Table 2). The majority (91.1%) of patients with a blood transfusion index above 2000 did not require autologous blood transfusion. By comparison, an autologous blood transfusion was required by 74.0% of those with a blood transfusion index below 2000. These figures included patients who did not undergo preoperative blood collection because of conditions such as acute aortic dissection.

## Discussion

Preoperative blood collection using rHuEPO combined with iron sulfate significantly reduced the requirement for autologous transfusion in thoracic aortic surgery. In this study, 84.4% of patients having elective thoracic aortic surgery did not require autologous blood transfusion. In the emergency cases, however, this was only the case for 48.1% of patients. One possible reason is that blood was not collected preoperatively from the emergency patients. Also, patients requiring emergency surgery sometimes have massive bleeding as the result of aneurysm rupture or cardiac tamponade.

TABLE 2

**Surgical information and postoperative course**

|  | N group (n = 40) | T group (n = 19) | p value |
|---|---|---|---|
| CPB time (min) | 190.9 ± 57.6 | 219.1 ± 73.5 | NS |
| Cardiac arrest time (min) | 111.2 ± 43.3 | 105.2 ± 44.0 | NS |
| Lowest rectal temperature | 23.7° ± 8.3° | 20.3° ± 4.5° | NS |
| Circulatory arrest (min) | 44.3 ± 23.6 | 45.2 ± 43.3 | NS |
| Bleeding, 12 hour (mL) | 320 ± 273 | 546 ± 367 | < 0.05 |
| Urine output, 12 hour (mL) | 1788 ± 763 | 1673 ± 632 | NS |
| Returned to operating theater for bleeding (patients) | 1 | 1 | NS |
| Mortality (%) | 5.0 | 26.3 | < 0.01 |

N group, patients not receiving blood transfusion; T group, patients receiving blood transfusion; NS, not significant

In coronary surgery, about 80% of patients do not require autologous blood transfusion.[23] Nevertheless, I consider that blood should be collected preoperatively from patients with a blood transfusion index below 2000. However, it should be appreciated that collecting blood preoperatively has cost and time implications.[24]

Finally, the blood transfusion index, which is easily determined from the multiplication of hematocrit and body weight, allows the transfusion requirement to be predicted.

### References

1. Shander A. Emerging risks and outcomes of blood transfusion in surgery. *Semin Hematol* 2004;41(1 suppl):117–24.

2. Goodnough LT, Shander A, Brecher ME. Transfusion medicine: looking to the future. *Lancet* 2003; 361:161–9.

3. Schroeder S, Borger N, Wrigge H et al. A tumor necrosis factor gene polymorphism influences the inflammatory response after cardiac operation. *Ann Thorac Surg* 2003;75:534–7.

4. Levy JH, Tanaka KA. Inflammatory response to cardiopulmonary bypass. *Ann Thorac Surg* 2003;75:715–20.

5. Mora Mangano CT, Neville MJ, Hsu PH. Aprotinin, blood loss, and renal dysfunction in deep hypothermic circulatory arrest. *Circulation* 2001;104(12suppl 1): I276–81.

6. Britton LW, Eastlund DT, Dziuban SW et al. Predonated autologous blood use in elective cardiac surgery. *Ann Thorac Surg* 1989;47:529–32.

7. Tyson GS, Sladen RN, Spainhour V et al. Blood conservation in cardiac surgery. Preliminary results with an institutional commitment. *Ann Surg* 1989;209:736–42.

8. Yoda M, Nonoyama M, Shimakura T et al. Preoperative autologous blood donation with cardiac surgery. *Kyobu Geka* 2003;56:479–82.

9. Kasper SM, Gerlich W, Buzello W. Preoperative red cell production in patients undergoing weekly autologous blood donation. *Transfusion* 1997;37:1058–62.

10. Kiyama H, Ohshima N, Imazeki T, Yamada T. Autologous blood donation with recombinant human erythropoietin in anemic patients. *Ann Thorac Surg* 1999;68:1652–6.

11. Oshima N, Kiyama H, Imazeki T. Combined erythropoietin and aprotinin use for blood conservation in elderly coronary bypass patients. *Kyobu Geka* 1997;50:707–10.

12. Hayashi J, Kumon K, Takanashi S. Subcutaneous administration of recombinant human erythropoietin before cardiac surgery: a double-blind, multicenter trial in Japan. *Transfusion* 1994;34:142–6.

13. Helm RE, Gold JP, Rosengart TK et al. Erythropoietin in cardiac surgery. *J Card Surg* 1993;8:579–606.

14. Ovrum E, Tangen G, Tollofsrud S, Ringold MA. Heparin-coated circuits and reduced systemic anticoagulation applied to 2500 consecutive first-time coronary artery bypass grafting procedures. *Ann Thorac Surg* 2003;76:1144–8.

15. Butler J, Murithi EW, Pathi VL et al. Duroflo II heparin bonding does not attenuate cytokine release or improve pulmonary function. *Ann Thorac Surg* 2002;74:139–42.

16. Mirow N, Brinkmann T, Minami K et al. Low dose systemic heparinization combined with heparin-coated extracorporeal circulation. Effects related to platelets. *J Cardiovasc Surg (Torino)* 2001;42:579–85.

17. Suenaga E, Naito K, Cao ZL et al. Experimental use of a compact centrifugal pump and membrane oxygenator as a cardiopulmonary support system. *Artif Organs* 2000;24:912–15.

18. Ikeda S, Johnston MF, Yagi K et al. Intraoperative autologous blood salvage with cardiac surgery: an analysis of five years' experience in more than 3,000 patients. *J Clin Anesth* 1992;4:359–66.

19. Costello JM, Backer CL, de Hoyos A. Aprotinin reduces operative closure time and blood product use after pediatric bypass. *Ann Thorac Surg* 2003;75:1261–6.

20. Mossinger H, Dietrich W, Braun SL et al. High-dose aprotinin reduces activation of hemostasis, allogeneic blood requirement, and duration of postoperative ventilation in pediatric cardiac surgery. *Ann Thorac Surg* 2003;75:430–7.

21. Landis RC, Asimakopoulos G, Poullis M et al. The antithrombotic and antiinflammatory mechanisms of action of aprotinin. *Ann Thorac Surg* 2001;72:2169–75.

22. Levy JH. Pharmacologic preservation of the hemostatic system during cardiac surgery. *Ann Thorac Surg* 2001;27:1814–20.

23. Suenaga E, Suda H, Katayama Y. Preoperative blood donation in coronary artery bypass grafting. *Jpn J Cardiovasc Surg* 2002;31:97–9.

24. Coyle D, Lee KM, Fergusson DA, Laupacis A. Cost effectiveness of epoetin-alpha to augment preoperative autologous blood donation in elective cardiac surgery. *Pharmacoeconomics* 2000;18:161–71.